INTRODUCTION

*Nourishing Blood Type
O - A Personal Journey
to Optimal Health*

Welcome to a journey of self-discovery, wellness, and empowerment. In the pages that follow, we delve into the fascinating realm of the Blood Type O diet, a personalised approach to nutrition that promises to unlock the potential of your unique biology. This isn't just another diet; it's a lifestyle designed to cater to your individual needs, and it might just be the missing piece in your pursuit of better health and vitality.

In the quest for a healthier and more fulfilling life, we often find ourselves overwhelmed by an abundance of dietary advice, fad diets, and conflicting information. What makes the Blood Type O diet unique is its foundation in the notion that our blood type holds vital clues to what our bodies truly need. Dr. Peter D'Adamo, the visionary mind behind this approach, suggests that understanding your blood type can revolutionise the way you eat and, consequently, the way you live.

In the chapters ahead, we will explore the fundamental principles of the blood type O diet and its potential to enhance your overall well-being. Whether you are just beginning to discover the concept or you're a seasoned practitioner, this book is a comprehensive guide to help you navigate the intricacies of the diet with confidence.

Our journey will encompass the essence of blood type O, delving into the unique characteristics and traits associated with this blood type. We will learn how to tailor our nutrition to better align with our genetic predispositions while considering the scientific foundations and the controversies that surround this approach.

We'll explore the primary dietary principles for blood type O, focusing on the role of proteins as the cornerstone of your nutrition. You'll discover the benefits of consuming specific fruits and vegetables and learn why some grains, legumes, and dairy products may not be your best allies in the quest for optimal health.

But this book is not just about theory. It's also a practical guide that provides you with tangible tools to make the blood type O diet work for you. You'll find meal plans, delicious recipes, and tips for easy implementation. We'll discuss the importance of hydration, the significance of healthy fats, and the role of exercise and lifestyle choices in your journey to better health.

Additionally, we'll share inspiring success stories from individuals who have embraced the Blood Type O diet, as well as insights into common challenges and how to overcome them.

This book is more than just a dietary guide; it's an invitation to embark on a personal journey of discovery and transformation. It's an opportunity to take charge of your health and well-being in a way that suits you uniquely. It's a chance to reconnect with the wisdom of your body, to honour its needs, and to nurture it with foods that can make a real difference.

So, are you ready to explore the world of blood type O nutrition, to embrace a diet that aligns with your blood type, and to take the first step towards lasting health and vitality? If so, turn the page, and let's begin this remarkable journey together.

CHAPTER 1:

Understanding Blood Type Diet

The Concept Of The Blood Type Diet

The concept of the blood type diet is a dietary theory that suggests an individual's blood type can play a significant role in determining what foods are most compatible with their genetic makeup. The theory was popularised by Dr. Peter D'Adamo in his book "Eat Right for Your Type," published in 1996. According to this theory, the foods you eat should be tailored to your specific blood type (A, B, AB, or O) to promote better health and well-being.

Here's an extensive explanation of the Blood Type Diet:

1. The Four Blood Types:

• Type A: This blood type is associated with agrarian or agricultural ancestors. It is often referred to as the "cultivator" blood type. People with type A blood are advised to follow a primarily plant-based diet, including fruits, vegetables, and grains, while avoiding or limiting animal products.

• Type B: This blood type is linked to nomadic ancestors and is called the "nomad" blood type. Individuals with type

B blood are recommended to have a balanced diet that includes a wide range of foods, such as meats, dairy, grains, and vegetables.

• Type AB: People with type AB blood are believed to have a more recent blend of type A and B traits. They are encouraged to eat a combination of foods suitable for both type A and type B.

• Type O: Type O is considered the "hunter" blood type, associated with early hunter-gatherer ancestors. Type O individuals are advised to consume a diet rich in animal protein, avoid grains and legumes, and focus on specific vegetables and fruits.

2. The Relationship Between Blood Type and Diet:

• According to the Blood Type Diet Theory, our blood type influences our susceptibility to certain illnesses and our ability to digest and metabolise specific foods. It is suggested that certain lectins (proteins found in foods) can react differently with each blood type, either promoting health or causing adverse reactions.

• For example, individuals with type O blood are believed to have a higher tolerance for meat and may benefit from a diet rich in animal protein. Type A individuals, on the other hand, are thought to have a more sensitive immune system and may do better with a vegetarian diet.

3. Key Dietary Guidelines:

• The diet emphasises the importance of avoiding "avoid foods" that are considered harmful for your blood type and consuming "beneficial foods" that are supportive of your blood type.

• Foods are categorised into four groups: "Highly

Beneficial," "Neutral," "Avoid," and "Not Well Tolerated."

• Dr. D'Adamo also considers other factors such as Rh factor and secretor status (whether you secrete your blood type antigens in bodily fluids) to further personalise dietary recommendations.

4. Exercise and Lifestyle:

• In addition to dietary recommendations, the Blood Type Diet includes suggestions for exercise and lifestyle choices. These recommendations are also tailored to an individual's blood type.

5. Critics and controversy:

• The Blood Type Diet has faced significant criticism from the scientific community. Many experts contend that the theory is unsupported by rigorous research and lacks scientific evidence.

• Numerous studies conducted to verify the diet's claims have yielded inconclusive results, and the theory remains largely anecdotal.

6. Personalisation and Individual Choices:

• While the Blood Type Diet has been widely criticised, some people report experiencing positive health changes when following its recommendations. As with any diet, individual experiences can vary.

How Does It Emerge?

Dr. Peter D'Adamo, a naturopathic doctor, popularized the

Blood Type Diet, also referred to as the "Eat Right for Your Type" diet, and it has its roots in the late 20th century. Here's a look at the origin, evolution, and creator of the Blood Type Diet:

Origin: The origin of the Blood Type Diet can be traced back to the publication of Dr. Peter D'Adamo's book, "Eat Right for Your Type," which was first published in 1996. Dr. D'Adamo's book introduced the concept that an individual's blood type could play a significant role in determining the optimal diet for their overall health and well-being. The book gained widespread attention and became a bestseller, leading to the diet's increased popularity.

Evolution: Over the years, the Blood Type Diet has evolved as Dr. D'Adamo continued to publish books and update his recommendations. He expanded his theory to include exercise and lifestyle guidelines tailored to specific blood types. The diet also includes considerations for an individual's Rh factor (positive or negative) and secretor status (whether one secretes blood-type antigens in bodily fluids like saliva).

Dr. D'Adamo has written several follow-up books, including "Cook Right for Your Type" and "Live Right for Your Type," which provide more detailed dietary and lifestyle recommendations based on an individual's blood type. These books further elaborated on the concept and aimed to help people make more informed choices.

Despite its early popularity, the Blood Type Diet has faced ongoing controversy and scepticism within the scientific and medical communities. Critics argue that the diet's claims lack robust scientific evidence, and studies attempting to validate its principles have yielded mixed results. As a result, the diet remains a subject of debate and caution.

The Creator: Dr. Peter D'Adamo, born on June 17, 1956, in Bridgeport, Connecticut, is the creator and main proponent of the Blood Type Diet. He comes from a family of naturopathic physicians, and he received his Doctor of Naturopathic Medicine degree from the National College of Naturopathic Medicine in 1982.

D'Adamo developed the Blood Type Diet based on his belief that an individual's blood type affects their dietary needs and susceptibility to various health conditions. He has written multiple books on the topic, presented his ideas at conferences, and conducted research to support his theories. However, his work has been met with significant criticism from the scientific community, as many have questioned the lack of rigorous scientific evidence to substantiate his claims.

Despite the controversies surrounding the Blood Type Diet, Dr. D'Adamo has maintained his advocacy for personalised nutrition based on blood type, and the diet continues to have a following among individuals who believe they have experienced positive health outcomes by following its recommendations. However, it's essential to approach this diet with a critical and informed perspective and consult with healthcare professionals for evidence-based dietary advice.

Individualised nutrition

The central premise of the Blood Type Diet is the focus on individualised nutrition based on an individual's blood type, specifically A, B, AB, or O, to promote better health and well-being.

Here's an explanation of how this concept works:

1. Blood Type Classification:

o There are four primary blood types: A, B, AB, and O. The presence or absence of specific antigens on the surface of red blood cells, such as the A, B, and Rh (Rhesus) factors, determines each blood type.

2. Dietary Recommendations by Blood Type:

o The diet suggests that each blood type has specific dietary requirements and intolerances based on their genetic makeup. This means that foods that are beneficial for one blood type may not be suitable for another.

o Dr. Peter D'Adamo, the creator of the Blood Type Diet, has developed a set of dietary guidelines and categorised foods into groups for each blood type:

■ Highly Beneficial Foods: These are foods that are considered optimal for a specific blood type, promoting health and well-being.

■ Neutral Foods: These foods are generally considered safe for consumption by all blood types.

■ Avoid foods: These are foods that should be strictly avoided as they may have adverse effects on health.

■ Not Well Tolerated Foods: These foods are not harmful but may not be optimal for a specific blood type.

3. Blood Type A:

o Individuals with blood type A are advised to follow a primarily plant-based diet rich in fruits, vegetables, and grains. They should limit or avoid animal products, particularly red meat.

4. Blood Type B:

o People with blood type B are encouraged to have a balanced diet that includes a variety of foods. This diet may include meats, dairy, grains, and vegetables.

5. Blood Type AB:

o Blood type: AB Individuals are recommended to consume a combination of foods suitable for both blood types A and B. Their diet should incorporate a variety of foods.

6. Blood Type O:

o Type O is advised to follow a diet that is rich in animal protein, especially lean meats. Grains and legumes should be limited, and certain fruits and vegetables should be emphasised.

7. Exercise and Lifestyle Considerations:

o In addition to dietary guidelines, the Blood Type Diet suggests that exercise and lifestyle choices should also be tailored to an individual's blood type. For example, certain blood types may benefit more from vigorous exercise, while others may thrive with relaxation techniques.

8. Rh Factor and Secretor Status:

o The Blood Type Diet also takes into account an individual's Rh factor (positive or negative) and secretor status, which can further refine dietary recommendations.

9. Controversy and Scepticism:

o The Blood Type Diet has faced significant criticism within the scientific and medical communities. Critics argue that the diet's claims lack robust scientific evidence, and studies attempting to validate its principles have yielded mixed results.

10. Individual experiences vary.

o Some individuals have reported positive health changes when following the blood type diet. However, it's essential to recognise that individual experiences can vary, and the diet's effectiveness remains a subject of debate and caution.

The Importance Of A Healthy Diet

A healthy diet plays a vital role in overall well-being, and it is particularly significant when considering the Blood Type Diet, with a focus on improving the health of individuals with Blood Type O. Here's why a healthy diet is essential for overall well-being, especially for those with blood type O:

1. Nutrient Balance: A healthy diet provides the essential nutrients, vitamins, and minerals that the body needs to function optimally. For Blood Type O individuals, a balanced diet ensures they receive the necessary nutrients that may be especially beneficial for their blood type.

2. Energy Levels: Proper nutrition ensures a steady and sustainable supply of energy, which is essential for physical and mental well-being. For blood type O, a diet that aligns with their blood type can help maintain energy levels and prevent fatigue.

3. Digestive Health: A healthy diet can support a well-functioning digestive system, which is crucial for nutrient absorption and overall health. Blood Type O individuals may benefit from a diet that minimises foods that could potentially lead to digestive discomfort.

4. Immune System Support: A nutritious diet can bolster the immune system, helping the body defend against illnesses and diseases. For individuals with blood type O, foods that are compatible with their blood type may contribute to a stronger immune response.

5. Weight Management: Maintaining a healthy weight is essential for overall well-being, as obesity can lead to various health issues. A diet that suits one's blood type may help with weight management and body composition.

6. Cardiovascular Health: Diet plays a critical role in cardiovascular health. A heart-healthy diet can help reduce the risk of heart disease, which is of particular concern for some blood type O individuals.

7. Inflammation Reduction: Certain foods can promote or reduce inflammation in the body. A diet that aligns with one's blood type may help reduce inflammation and lower the risk of chronic inflammatory conditions.

8. Improved Mental Health: The link between diet and mental health is well established. A balanced and nutrient-rich diet can have a positive impact on mood, cognitive function, and overall mental well-being.

9. Prevention of Chronic Diseases: A healthy diet is a key factor in preventing chronic diseases such as diabetes, hypertension, and certain types of cancer. Dietary choices tailored to one's blood type may contribute to disease prevention.

10. Longevity and Quality of Life: Eating well is associated with a longer, healthier life. For individuals with blood type O, adhering to a diet that aligns with their blood type may enhance their overall quality of life and longevity.

CHAPTER 2:

Understanding Blood Type O

An Overview Of Blood Types

Blood types are classifications of blood based on the presence or absence of specific antigens on the surface of red blood cells. The two most critical blood group systems are the ABO system and the Rh factor.

Here's an overview of blood types and the main blood group systems:

1. ABO Blood Group System:

• The ABO blood group system is the most well-known and widely used blood typing system. It categorises blood into four main groups: A, B, AB, and O, based on the presence or absence of two antigens, A and B.

• Each person inherits one ABO gene from each parent, resulting in the following possible combinations:

o Type A has A antigens on the red blood cells and B antibodies in the plasma.

o Type B has B antigens on the red blood cells and A antibodies in the plasma.

o Type AB: Has both A and B antigens on the red blood cells and no A or B antibodies in the plasma. This is known as the universal recipient blood type.

o Type O: Has no A or B antigens on the red blood cells and both A and B antibodies in the plasma. This is known as the universal donor blood type.

2. Rh Factor (Rhesus Factor):

• The Rh factor is another crucial component of blood typing. It is either present (+) or absent (-) on the surface of red blood cells. A person who has the Rh factor is said to be Rh-positive, while a person without it is Rh-negative.

• When ABO blood type and Rh factor are combined, it results in eight primary blood types, including A+, A-, B+, B-, AB+, AB-, O+, and O-. For example, A+ indicates a blood type A person with the Rh factor, while O- indicates a blood type O person without the Rh factor.

3. Other blood group systems:

• In addition to the ABO and Rh systems, there are numerous other blood group systems with various antigens. These systems are less well-known but can be critical in specific medical situations. Some of these systems include the Kell, Duffy, Kidd, Lewis, and P systems, among others.

Blood Transfusions And Compatibility:

• Blood type compatibility is crucial in medical situations involving blood transfusions or organ transplantation. Incompatible blood transfusions can lead to severe reactions and health complications.

• For safe blood transfusions, it's essential to match the ABO and Rh blood types between the donor and the recipient. For example, a person with type A+ blood can receive blood from type A+ or type O+ donors, but not from type B+ or AB + donors.

• Rh-negative individuals should receive Rh-negative blood, while Rh-positive individuals can receive Rh-negative or Rh-positive blood.

Blood Typing and Genetic Inheritance:

• The alleles that a person inherits from their parents play a role in determining their blood type. For example, a child with two A alleles (AA) will have blood type A, while a child with one A allele and one B allele (AB) will have blood type AB.

• Blood type inheritance follows Mendelian genetics, and the specific combination of alleles determines the ABO blood group and Rh factor.

Blood Type O

Blood Type O is one of the four primary blood types in the ABO blood group system, the other three being A, B, and AB. Blood Type O is characterised by the absence of both A and B antigens on the surface of red blood cells. Here's an overview of blood type O and some of its key characteristics:

Blood Type O Characteristics:

1. Universal Donor: Blood Type O is often referred to as the

"universal donor" because individuals with this blood type can donate red blood cells to people of any other blood type (A, B, AB, or O). This is because blood type O has neither A nor B antigens on the surface of its red blood cells, making it less likely to trigger an immune response in the recipient.

2. Recipient Compatibility: People with blood type O can receive blood only from other blood type O individuals. This restriction is due to the presence of both anti-A and anti-B antibodies in the plasma of Blood Type O individuals, which can react against A or B antigens in the donor blood.

3. Rh Factor Compatibility: Blood Type O can be either Rh-positive (O+) or Rh-negative (O-), depending on the presence or absence of the Rh factor (Rhesus factor). For example, O+ means that the individual is blood type O with the Rh factor, while O- means that the individual is blood type O without the Rh factor.

4. Compatibility with Platelets and Plasma: Blood Type O individuals may also have specific plasma and platelet compatibility considerations, but these are not as widely emphasised as ABO and Rh compatibility.

5. Traits Associated with Blood Type O: The Blood Type Diet suggests that individuals with Blood Type O may have certain traits and dietary recommendations. This includes a focus on high-protein diets, the avoidance of certain grains and legumes, and an emphasis on specific fruits and vegetables.

6. Health Considerations: Some studies have suggested potential associations between blood type and various health conditions. For instance, some research has explored links between blood type and susceptibility

to certain diseases, such as heart disease and certain infections, although these associations are generally not considered strong enough to be used for clinical diagnosis or treatment.

7. Population Distribution: The distribution of blood types in the population varies by region and ethnicity. Blood type O is the most common blood type in many parts of the world, including Asia.

The Characteristics And Traits Associated With Blood Type O Individuals

The Blood Type Diet, developed by Dr. Peter D'Adamo, suggests that individuals with Blood Type O have specific characteristics and traits and that their dietary and lifestyle recommendations should be tailored to these traits. It's important to note that the validity and scientific support for these claims are widely debated, and many experts consider them to be largely anecdotal. Here are some of the characteristics and traits associated with blood type O individuals according to the blood type diet theory:

1. Strength and resilience:

• Blood Type O individuals are often described as strong and robust. They are believed to have inherited traits from their hunter-gatherer ancestors, which make them physically hardy and better suited to a high-protein, meat-based diet.

2. High energy levels:

• Blood Type O individuals are said to have naturally high energy levels and can handle rigorous physical activity better than other blood types. As a result, exercise and physical activity are emphasised in their lifestyle recommendations.

3. Strong Digestive System:

• The Blood Type Diet suggests that people with Blood Type O have a robust digestive system, especially when it comes to digesting animal proteins. They are believed to produce ample stomach acid and enzymes to break down meat efficiently.

4. Prone to stress:

• Blood Type O individuals are often described as being more prone to stress and can experience heightened levels of the stress hormone cortisol. Stress management techniques are recommended to help mitigate these effects.

5. Increased Risk of Certain Health Issues:

• According to the Blood Type Diet Theory, individuals with blood type O may be more susceptible to certain health issues, such as ulcers, thyroid problems, and autoimmune diseases. To mitigate these risks, dietary and lifestyle adjustments are proposed.

6. Favourable Foods:

• The diet recommends a high-protein diet for Blood Type O individuals, with a focus on lean meats, fish, and poultry. Specific vegetables and fruits are also suggested to be beneficial. Dairy, grains, and legumes are often discouraged or limited.

7. Potential for Weight Loss:

• Blood Type O individuals are thought to have a higher metabolic rate, making it easier for them to lose weight and maintain a healthy body composition when following the recommended diet.

8. Intolerance to Certain Foods:

• The Blood Type Diet suggests that Blood Type O individuals may have adverse reactions to certain foods, particularly wheat products, due to the presence of lectins that interact negatively with their blood type.

CHAPTER 3:

The Blood Type O Diet Basics

Based on Dr. Peter D'Adamo's Blood Type Diet theory, the Blood Type O Diet makes specific dietary suggestions for people with Blood Type O. These recommendations are said to be tailored to the genetic traits associated with blood type O. Keep in mind that the scientific support for these recommendations is limited, and the diet remains a subject of controversy. However, here are the key essentials of the Blood Type O Diet:

1. Emphasis on Protein:

• The Blood Type O Diet places a strong emphasis on the consumption of animal protein, particularly lean meats like poultry, fish, and red meat. Protein is considered a key component of this diet.

2. Meat and seafood:

• High-protein animal sources such as beef, lamb, venison, turkey, chicken, and fish are encouraged. Dr. D'Adamo suggests that people with blood type O may digest these proteins more efficiently.

3. Limited Grains:

• The diet recommends limited consumption of grains, particularly wheat products. It suggests that certain lectins found in wheat can be detrimental to blood type O individuals.

4. Legumes:

• Legumes, such as lentils, beans, and peanuts, are often discouraged or limited. These foods are believed to be less compatible with blood type O.

5. Fruits and vegetables:

• The diet suggests specific fruits and vegetables that are considered beneficial for blood type O individuals. These may include leafy greens, sweet potatoes, and certain fruits like berries and plums.

6. Dairy Products:

• The Blood Type O Diet recommends limiting or avoiding dairy products, as they are thought to be less compatible with this blood type.

7. Healthy Fats:

• Healthy fats, such as olive oil and flaxseed oil, are encouraged. These fats are believed to support overall health.

8. Exercise and stress reduction:

• The diet includes lifestyle recommendations, such as engaging in regular, vigorous exercise, as well as stress management techniques, to help maintain health and well-being for Blood Type O individuals.

9. Avoid processed foods.

• Highly processed and refined foods should be avoided.

Fresh, whole, and unprocessed foods are promoted.

10. Portion Control and Meal Timing: The diet suggests eating smaller, more frequent meals and avoiding late-night meals for better digestion and metabolism.

11. Limit Caffeine and Alcohol: The consumption of coffee, black tea, and alcohol is often recommended in moderation for blood type O individuals.

12. Individual Variations: The Blood Type Diet also takes into account individual variations within the blood type, considering factors such as secretor status (whether you secrete blood type antigens in bodily fluids) and the Rh factor.

The Primary Dietary Principles For Blood Type O

The primary dietary principles for individuals with Blood Type O, according to the Blood Type Diet Theory, emphasise specific food choices and lifestyle recommendations tailored to their blood type. These recommendations are designed to optimise health and well-being based on the genetic traits associated with blood type O. It's important to note that the scientific support for these principles is limited, and the diet remains a subject of controversy.

However, here are the key dietary principles for blood type O:

1. High-Protein Diet:

• Blood Type O individuals are encouraged to consume a high-protein diet, particularly focusing on lean animal sources. This includes poultry, fish, lean cuts of red meat, and game meats.

2. Limit Grains:

• Grains, particularly those containing wheat products, are generally discouraged or limited for blood type O individuals. It is believed that the lectins in certain grains may be less compatible with their blood type.

3. Emphasis on Vegetables:

• The diet recommends an abundance of vegetables, particularly leafy greens. Vegetables are a primary source of essential nutrients, fibre, and antioxidants.

4. Select Fruits:

• Specific fruits like berries, plums, and figs are considered beneficial for blood type O individuals. These fruits are believed to support their health.

5. Limit Legumes:

• Legumes, such as beans, lentils, and peanuts, are often discouraged or recommended in moderation, as they are thought to have lectins that may not be well-tolerated.

6. Dairy Moderation:

• Dairy products are typically recommended in moderation or limited amounts, as they may not be as compatible with blood type O.

7. Healthy Fats:

• Healthy fats from sources like olive oil, flaxseed oil, and nuts are encouraged for overall well-being.

8. Avoid processed foods.

• Highly processed and refined foods should be avoided, while fresh, whole, and unprocessed foods are promoted.

9. Portion Control:

• The diet suggests eating smaller, more frequent meals. This can help maintain stable energy levels and manage weight.

10. Hydration: Staying well-hydrated is important for all blood types. Drinking plenty of water and avoiding sugary or artificial beverages is recommended.

11. Avoid Certain Foods: Foods to be avoided by Blood Type O individuals include corn, cabbage, Brussels sprouts, and other specific items thought to be less compatible with their blood type.

12. Caffeine and Alcohol Moderation: Consumption of coffee, black tea, and alcohol is often recommended in moderation for blood type O individuals.

13. Regular Exercise: Vigorous physical activity is emphasised for Blood Type O individuals to maintain their energy levels and overall health.

14. Stress Management: Stress management techniques, such as meditation or relaxation exercises, are suggested to help mitigate the impact of stress, which Blood Type O individuals are believed to be more prone to.

What To Eat And Avoid

According to the Blood Type Diet Theory, individuals with Blood Type O are encouraged to eat specific foods that are considered beneficial for their blood type and to avoid or limit foods that are believed to be less compatible.

Keep in mind that the scientific support for these recommendations is limited, and the diet is controversial.

However, here is a general guideline on what to eat and what to avoid for Blood Type O individuals:

Foods To Eat (Beneficial Foods):

1. High-Quality Protein:

o Lean cuts of beef, lamb, venison, and other red meats

o Poultry, such as turkey and chicken.

o Fish, particularly deep-sea and cold-water varieties like salmon and mackerel

2. Fruits:

o Berries, including blueberries, blackberries, and strawberries

o Plums, figs, and prunes

o Apples and pears

3. Vegetables:

o Leafy greens, like spinach and kale,

o Broccoli, cauliflower, and Brussels sprouts

o Sweet potatoes and yams

4. Healthy Fats:

o Olive oil and flaxseed oil

o Nuts and seeds, including walnuts and flaxseeds

5. Beverages:

o Herbal teas, green tea, and red wine (in moderation).

Foods To Avoid Or Limit (Avoid Foods):

1. Grains:

o Wheat and wheat-based products, including bread and pasta.

o Corn and corn-based products.

2. Legumes:

o Beans, lentils, and peanuts.

3. Dairy Products:

o Cow's milk, particularly whole milk.

o Cheese, except for feta and mozzarella in moderation.

o Cottage cheese and other dairy-based products

4. Certain Vegetables:

o Brussels sprouts, cabbage, and cauliflower

o Eggplant and mushrooms

5. Fruits:

o Oranges and orange juice

6. Processed and artificial foods:

o Highly processed and artificial foods, including sugary snacks and artificial additives.

7. Beverages:

o Coffee and black tea.

8. Alcohol:

o Alcohol should be consumed in moderation, with red

wine being the preferred choice.

Food Recommendations

The Blood Type Diet suggests specific food recommendations for individuals with Blood Type O, emphasizing foods that are believed to be beneficial for this blood type. Keep in mind that the scientific support for these recommendations is limited, and the diet is controversial. Here are some food recommendations for blood type O individuals, with examples:

1. High-Quality Protein:

• Beneficial Foods: Lean meats and poultry are recommended for their high protein content.

• Examples:

o Lean beef (e.g., sirloin, tenderloin)

o Turkey breast

o Skinless chicken

o Lamb

2. Fish:

• Beneficial Foods: Cold-water and deep-sea fish are encouraged for their protein and omega-3 fatty acids.

• Examples:

o Salmon

o Mackerel

o Cod

o Trout

o Haddock

3. Fruits:

• Beneficial Foods: Certain fruits are recommended for blood type O individuals.

• Examples:

o Blueberries

o Blackberries

o Strawberries

o Plums

o Cherries

4. Vegetables:

• Beneficial Foods: Leafy greens and cruciferous vegetables are often emphasised.

• Examples:

o Spinach

o Kale

o Broccoli

o Brussels sprouts

o Collard greens

5. Healthy Fats:

• Beneficial Foods: Monounsaturated fats from olive oil and flaxseed oil are recommended.

• Examples:

o Extra virgin olive oil

o Flaxseed oil

6. Nuts and seeds:

• Beneficial Foods: Nuts and seeds are encouraged, particularly walnuts and flaxseeds.

• Examples:

o Walnuts

o Flaxseeds

o Almonds (in moderation)

7. Herbs and Spices:

• Beneficial Foods: Some herbs and spices can be incorporated into the diet.

• Examples:

o Garlic

o Ginger

o Turmeric

o Parsley

8. Beverages:

• Beneficial Foods: Herbal teas and green tea are often suggested.

• Examples:

o Green tea

o Peppermint tea

o Chamomile tea

9. Alcohol:

• Beneficial Foods: Red wine is recommended in moderation for its potential health benefits.

• Examples:

o High-quality red wine (in moderation)

10. Water: Staying well-hydrated is essential for all blood types. Drinking plain water is recommended.

CHAPTER 4

High-Quality Protein:

Grilled Sirloin Steak with Garlic Herb Butter

Ingredients:

- 1 lean sirloin steak (6–8 oz)

- 2 cloves of garlic, minced

- 1 tablespoon of fresh rosemary, chopped

- 1 tablespoon of fresh thyme, chopped

- 2 tablespoons of grass-fed butter or ghee

- Salt and freshly ground black pepper, to taste

Instructions:

For the garlic herb butter:

1. Start by preparing the garlic herb butter. In a small bowl, combine the minced garlic, chopped rosemary, and thyme.

2. In a saucepan over low heat, melt the grass-fed butter or ghee. Once melted, add the garlic and herb mixture. Sauté for about 1-2 minutes until the garlic becomes fragrant. Remove from heat and set aside.

3. Transfer the garlic herb butter to a piece of plastic wrap, roll it into a log, and refrigerate for at least 30 minutes to allow it to solidify.

For the Grilled Sirloin Steak:

1. Preheat your grill to medium-high heat (about 400–450°F or 200–230°C).

2. While the grill is heating, remove the sirloin steak from the refrigerator and let it sit at room temperature for about 20–30 minutes. This ensures even cooking.

3. Season the steak with salt and freshly ground black pepper on both sides.

4. Once the grill is hot, place the seasoned sirloin steak on the grill. Grill for about 4-5 minutes per side for medium-rare, or adjust the cooking time to your desired level of doneness.

5. While grilling, you can baste the steak with some of the prepared garlic herb butter. This will infuse the steak with additional flavour.

6. When the steak reaches your preferred doneness, remove it from the grill and allow it to rest for a few minutes. Resting the steak ensures the juices redistribute, resulting in a juicier, more tender steak.

7. Slice the steak against the grain, and serve it with a pat of the garlic herb butter on top. You can also drizzle any remaining garlic and herb butter over the steak for added flavour.

Nutritional Information (approximate):

• Serving Size: 1 steak with garlic herb butter

• Calories: 350-400 kcal

• Protein: 30-35g

• Fat: 25-30g

• Carbohydrates: 1g

• Fibre: 0g

• Sugars: 0g

• Cholesterol: 80-100mg

• Sodium: 300-400mg

Mediterranean Turkey and Vegetable Skewers

Ingredients:

• 1 pound of turkey breast, cut into chunks

• 2 bell peppers (red, yellow, or green), cut into chunks

• 2 small zucchinis, sliced into rounds

• 1 red onion, cut into chunks

• 2 tablespoons of extra virgin olive oil

• 1 teaspoon of dried Mediterranean herbs and spices (e.g., oregano, basil, thyme)

• Salt and freshly ground black pepper, to taste

• Wooden skewers, soaked in water for 30 minutes

Instructions:

1. Begin by marinating the turkey. In a bowl, combine the turkey chunks, extra virgin olive oil, dried Mediterranean herbs and spices, salt, and freshly ground black pepper. Toss to coat the turkey pieces evenly. Allow the turkey to marinate for at least 30 minutes in the refrigerator.

2. While the turkey is marinating, prepare the vegetables. Cut the bell peppers, zucchinis, and red onion into chunks or rounds, making sure they are roughly the same size for even cooking.

3. Preheat your grill to medium-high heat (about 400–450°F or 200–230°C).

4. Assemble the skewers by alternately threading the marinated turkey chunks and the prepared vegetables onto the soaked wooden skewers. Ensure the skewers are well-balanced with a combination of turkey and vegetables.

5. Brush the skewers with a little extra olive oil to prevent sticking to the grill grates.

6. Place the skewers on the preheated grill and cook for about 4-6 minutes per side, or until the turkey is cooked through and the vegetables are tender and slightly charred.

7. Keep a close eye on the skewers and turn them as needed to ensure even cooking.

8. Once the turkey is cooked, remove the skewers from the grill. Allow them to rest for a couple of minutes.

9. Serve the Mediterranean Turkey and Vegetable Skewers hot, garnished with a little extra dried herbs and spices if desired.

Nutritional Information (approximate):

• Serving Size: 1 skewer

• Calories: 150–170 kcal

• Protein: 20-25g

• Fat: 4-6g

• Carbohydrates: 7-10g

• Fibre: 2-3g

• Sugars: 4-6g

• Cholesterol: 50-70mg

• Sodium: 40-60mg

Lemon Herb Chicken Salad

Ingredients:

• 2 boneless, skinless chicken breasts or thighs

• Juice of 1-2 fresh lemons (about 1/4 cup)

• 2 tablespoons of extra virgin olive oil

• 2 tablespoons of fresh herbs (e.g., parsley, cilantro), finely chopped

• Salt and freshly ground black pepper, to taste

• Mixed greens (e.g., spinach, arugula, romaine lettuce)

• Assorted vegetables (e.g., cherry tomatoes, cucumber, red onion)

Instructions:

For the Lemon Herb Marinade:

1. In a bowl, combine the fresh lemon juice, extra virgin olive oil, and the chopped fresh herbs (parsley and cilantro). Mix well to create the marinade.

2. Season the marinade with a pinch of salt and freshly ground black pepper, adjusting to taste.

3. Set aside a small portion of the marinade for later use as a salad dressing.

4. Place the chicken breasts or thighs in a shallow dish or a resealable plastic bag, and pour the remaining marinade over them.

5. Seal the bag or cover the dish and refrigerate for at least 30 minutes (or up to 4 hours) to allow the chicken to marinate and absorb the flavours.

For grilling the chicken:

1. Preheat your grill to medium-high heat (about 400–450°F or 200–230°C).

2. Once the grill is hot, remove the chicken from the marinade, allowing any excess to drip off. Discard the marinade used for the chicken.

3. Grill the chicken for about 6–8 minutes per side, or until it's no longer pink in the centre and the internal temperature reaches 165°F (75°C).

4. Transfer the grilled chicken to a plate and allow it to rest for a few minutes. Then, slice it into thin strips.

Assembling the Salad:

1. In a large bowl, combine the mixed greens and assorted vegetables (e.g., cherry tomatoes, cucumber, and red onion).

2. Drizzle the reserved marinade over the salad and toss to coat the greens and veggies.

3. Add the sliced lemon herb chicken on top of the salad.

4. Garnish with additional fresh herbs and a wedge of lemon, if desired.

Nutritional Information (approximate):

• Serving Size: 1/4 of the recipe (with 1 chicken breast)

• Calories: 250–300 kcal

• Protein: 25-30g

• Fat: 15-20g

• Carbohydrates: 10-15g

• Fibre: 2-3g

- Sugars: 3-4g
- Cholesterol: 70-90mg
- Sodium: 200-250mg

Balsamic-glazed lamb chops

Ingredients:

- 4 lamb chops (about 1 inch thick)
- 1/4 cup balsamic vinegar
- 2 cloves of garlic, minced
- 1 tablespoon of fresh rosemary, chopped
- 1 tablespoon of Dijon mustard
- Salt and freshly ground black pepper, to taste
- Olive oil for cooking

Instructions:

For the balsamic glaze:

1. In a small saucepan over medium heat, combine the balsamic vinegar, minced garlic, and fresh rosemary.

2. Bring the mixture to a simmer and let it cook for about 5-7 minutes, or until it has reduced by half and thickened.

3. Remove the saucepan from the heat and whisk in the Dijon mustard. Season with a pinch of salt and freshly ground black pepper. Set the glaze aside.

For the lamb chops:

1. Season the lamb chops with salt and freshly ground black pepper on both sides.

2. Preheat a skillet or grill pan over medium-high heat and

add a little olive oil to prevent sticking.

3. Place the seasoned lamb chops in the hot skillet or grill pan and cook for about 4-5 minutes per side for medium-rare, or adjust the cooking time to your desired level of doneness.

4. During the last few minutes of cooking, brush the lamb chops with the prepared balsamic glaze, ensuring they are coated evenly.

5. Once the lamb chops are cooked to your liking, remove them from the heat and let them rest for a couple of minutes.

For Serving:

1. Drizzle any remaining balsamic glaze over the lamb chops before serving.

2. Garnish with additional fresh rosemary, if desired.

Nutritional Information (approximate):

• Serving Size: 1 lamb chop with balsamic glaze

• Calories: 250–300 kcal

• Protein: 25-30g

• Fat: 15-20g

• Carbohydrates: 6-8g

• Fibre: 1g

• Sugars: 5-7g

• Cholesterol: 75-95mg

• Sodium: 150-200mg

Grilled Salmon with Dill Sauce

Ingredients:

• 4 salmon fillets (6–8 oz each)

• 2 tablespoons of fresh dill, finely chopped

• Juice of 1 lemon (about 2 tablespoons)

• 1/2 cup of Greek yoghurt or a dairy-free alternative

• 2 cloves of garlic, minced

• Salt and freshly ground black pepper, to taste

• Olive oil for grilling

Instructions:

For the Dill Sauce:

1. In a small bowl, combine the Greek yoghurt (or dairy-free alternative), minced garlic, fresh dill, and lemon juice. Mix well to create the dill sauce.

2. Season the sauce with a pinch of salt and freshly ground black pepper, adjusting to taste. Refrigerate the sauce until the salmon is ready to serve.

For grilling the salmon:

1. Preheat your grill to medium-high heat (about 400–450°F or 200–230°C).

2. While the grill is heating, brush the salmon fillets lightly with olive oil to prevent sticking.

3. Season the salmon fillets with salt and freshly ground black pepper.

4. Place the seasoned salmon fillets on the hot grill grates and cook for about 4-6 minutes per side, or until the salmon is cooked through and flakes easily with a fork.

5. Keep a close eye on the fillets and turn them as needed to

ensure even cooking.

6. Once the salmon is cooked to your liking, remove it from the grill and allow it to rest for a few minutes.

For Serving:

1. Serve the grilled salmon hot, with a generous drizzle of the prepared dill sauce on top.

2. Garnish with additional fresh dill and lemon wedges, if desired.

Nutritional Information (approximate):

• Serving Size: 1 salmon fillet with dill sauce

• Calories: 300–350 kcal

• Protein: 30-35g

• Fat: 15-20g

• Carbohydrates: 6-8g

• Fibre: 1g

• Sugars: 3-4g

• Cholesterol: 70-90mg

• Sodium: 150-200mg

CHAPTER 5

Fish:

Grilled Salmon with Lemon and Dill

Ingredients:

• 4 salmon fillets (6–8 oz each)

• Juice of 2 lemons (about 1/4 cup)

• 2 tablespoons of fresh dill, finely chopped

• 2 cloves of garlic, minced

• 2 tablespoons of olive oil

• Salt and freshly ground black pepper, to taste

Instructions:

For the Marinade:

1. In a small bowl, combine the fresh lemon juice, minced garlic, fresh dill, and olive oil. Mix well to create the marinade.

2. Season the marinade with a pinch of salt and freshly ground black pepper, adjusting to taste.

3. Place the salmon fillets in a shallow dish or a resealable plastic bag, and pour the marinade over them.

4. Seal the bag or cover the dish and refrigerate for at least 30 minutes to allow the salmon to marinate and absorb the

flavors. You can marinate for longer if you prefer a more intense flavour.

For grilling the salmon:

1. Preheat your grill to medium-high heat (about 400–450°F or 200–230°C).

2. While the grill is heating, brush the salmon fillets lightly with olive oil to prevent sticking.

3. Season the salmon fillets with a touch of salt and freshly ground black pepper.

4. Place the marinated salmon fillets on the hot grill grates and cook for about 4-6 minutes per side, or until the salmon is cooked through and flakes easily with a fork.

5. Keep a close eye on the fillets and turn them as needed to ensure even cooking.

6. Once the salmon is cooked to your liking, remove it from the grill and let it rest for a few minutes.

For Serving:

1. Serve the grilled salmon hot, with an optional garnish of additional fresh dill and lemon wedges.

Nutritional Information (approximate):

• Serving Size: 1 salmon fillet

• Calories: 300–350 kcal

• Protein: 30-35g

• Fat: 15-20g

• Carbohydrates: 6-8g

• Fibre: 1g

• Sugars: 1-2g

• Cholesterol: 70-90mg

• Sodium: 150-200mg

Mackerel Salad with Avocado and Arugula

Ingredients:

• 2 mackerel fillets

• 1 ripe avocado, sliced

• 2 cups of fresh arugula

• 2 tablespoons of extra virgin olive oil

• 1 tablespoon of fresh lemon juice

• 1 teaspoon of Dijon mustard

• Salt and freshly ground black pepper, to taste

Instructions:

For the dressing:

1. In a small bowl, prepare the dressing by whisking together the extra virgin olive oil, fresh lemon juice, and Dijon mustard. Season with a pinch of salt and freshly ground black pepper to taste. Set the dressing aside.

For Grilling the Mackerel:

1. Preheat your grill to medium-high heat (about 400–450°F or 200–230°C).

2. While the grill is heating, brush the mackerel fillets lightly with olive oil to prevent sticking.

3. Season the fillets with a touch of salt and freshly ground black pepper.

4. Place the mackerel fillets on the hot grill grates and cook

for about 4-6 minutes per side, or until the fish is cooked through and flakes easily with a fork.

5. Keep a close eye on the fillets and turn them as needed to ensure even cooking.

6. Once the mackerel is cooked to your liking, remove it from the grill and let it rest for a few minutes.

Assembling the Salad:

1. In a large salad bowl, combine the fresh arugula and sliced avocado.

2. Drizzle the prepared dressing over the arugula and avocado. Toss to coat the salad ingredients evenly.

3. Once the mackerel fillets have rested, flake the fish into chunks using a fork.

For Serving:

1. Arrange the flaked mackerel on top of the arugula and avocado salad.

2. Optionally, garnish with a drizzle of extra dressing and a sprinkle of fresh lemon zest or herbs for added flavour.

Nutritional Information (approximate):

• Serving Size: 1/2 of the salad with mackerel

• Calories: 300–350 kcal

• Protein: 20-25g

• Fat: 20-25g

• Carbohydrates: 10-15g

• Fibre: 6-8g

• Sugars: 1-2g

• Cholesterol: 60-80mg

• Sodium: 200-250mg

Baked Cod with Herbed Tomatoes

Ingredients:

• 4 cod fillets (6–8 oz each)

• 4 medium-sized fresh tomatoes, diced

• 1/4 cup of fresh basil, chopped

• 4 cloves of garlic, minced

• 2 tablespoons of extra virgin olive oil

• 1 teaspoon of dried oregano

• Salt and freshly ground black pepper, to taste

Instructions:

For the herb tomato topping:

1. In a mixing bowl, combine the diced tomatoes, minced garlic, chopped fresh basil, and dried oregano. Mix well to create the herbed tomato topping.

2. Season the topping with a pinch of salt and freshly ground black pepper, adjusting to taste. Set the toppings aside.

For baking the cod:

1. Preheat your oven to 375°F (190°C).

2. Place the cod fillets in a baking dish that has been lightly greased with olive oil to prevent sticking.

3. Drizzle a bit of olive oil over the cod fillets and season them with salt and freshly ground black pepper.

4. Spoon the herbed tomato topping over the cod fillets, ensuring an even distribution.

5. Cover the baking dish with aluminium foil.

6. Bake in the preheated oven for about 20–25 minutes, or until the cod is opaque and easily flakes with a fork.

7. Remove the foil and bake for an additional 5 minutes to allow the topping to lightly brown.

For Serving:

1. Serve the baked cod with herbed tomatoes hot, garnished with extra fresh basil if desired.

Nutritional Information (approximate):

• Serving Size: 1 cod fillet with herbed tomatoes

• Calories: 200-250 kcal

• Protein: 20-25g

• Fat: 6-8g

• Carbohydrates: 8-10g

• Fibre: 2-3g

• Sugars: 4-6g

• Cholesterol: 50-70mg

• Sodium: 100-150mg

Trout Almondine

Ingredients:

• 4 trout fillets

• 1/2 cup slivered almonds

• Juice of 1 lemon (about 2 tablespoons)

• 4 tablespoons of butter or ghee

• 2 tablespoons of fresh parsley, chopped

• Salt and freshly ground black pepper, to taste

Instructions:

For the almond sauce:

1. In a small saucepan over medium heat, melt the butter or ghee.

2. Add the slivered almonds to the melted butter and cook, stirring frequently, until the almonds turn a golden brown colour and become fragrant. This should take about 3–5 minutes.

3. Remove the saucepan from the heat and stir in the lemon juice. Season the sauce with a pinch of salt and freshly ground black pepper, to taste. Set the almondine sauce aside.

For pan-frying the trout:

1. Season the trout fillets with a touch of salt and freshly ground black pepper.

2. In a large skillet, heat a little butter or ghee over medium-high heat.

3. Place the seasoned trout fillets in the skillet and cook for about 2-3 minutes on each side, or until the fish is cooked through and the flesh flakes easily with a fork. The cooking time may vary based on the thickness of the fillets.

For Serving:

1. Drizzle the prepared almondine sauce over the cooked trout fillets.

2. Garnish the dish with chopped, fresh parsley.

Nutritional Information (approximate):

• Serving Size: 1 trout fillet with almondine sauce

• Calories: 250–300 kcal

• Protein: 20-25g

• Fat: 15-20g

• Carbohydrates: 6-8g

• Fibre: 2-3g

• Sugars: 1-2g

• Cholesterol: 70-90mg

• Sodium: 150-200mg

Haddock with Garlic-Herb Butter and Asparagus

Ingredients:

• 4 haddock fillets

• 1 bunch of fresh asparagus, trimmed

• 4 cloves of garlic, minced

• 2 tablespoons of fresh herbs (e.g., thyme, rosemary), finely chopped

• 4 tablespoons of grass-fed butter or ghee

• Zest of 1 lemon

• Salt and freshly ground black pepper, to taste

Instructions:

For the garlic-herb butter:

1. In a small saucepan over medium heat, melt the grass-fed butter or ghee.

2. Add the minced garlic and chopped fresh herbs (thyme and rosemary) to the melted butter. Cook for a few minutes until the garlic is fragrant and the herbs have infused into the butter.

3. Remove the saucepan from the heat and stir in the lemon zest. Season the garlic-herb butter with a pinch of salt and freshly ground black pepper. Set it aside.

For baking the haddock and asparagus:

1. Preheat your oven to 375°F (190°C).

2. Arrange the trimmed asparagus in a single layer on a baking sheet.

3. Drizzle some of the prepared garlic-herb butter over the asparagus and toss to coat them evenly.

4. Season the asparagus with salt and freshly ground black pepper.

5. Place the haddock fillets on the baking sheet beside the asparagus.

6. Drizzle the remaining garlic-herb butter over the haddock fillets, ensuring they are well coated.

7. Season the haddock with salt and freshly ground black pepper.

8. Bake in the preheated oven for about 15-20 minutes or until the haddock is opaque and flakes easily with a fork, and the asparagus is tender but still crisp.

For Serving:

1. Serve the haddock with garlic-herb butter and asparagus hot, with an optional garnish of additional lemon zest and

fresh herbs.

Nutritional Information (approximate):

• Serving Size: 1 haddock fillet with asparagus

• Calories: 250–300 kcal

• Protein: 25-30g

• Fat: 15-20g

• Carbohydrates: 8-10g

• Fibre: 4-6g

• Sugars: 2-3g

• Cholesterol: 75-95mg

• Sodium: 250-300mg

CHAPTER 6.

Fruits:

Berry Breakfast Parfait

Ingredients:

- 1 cup of fresh blueberries

- 1 cup of fresh blackberries

- 1 cup of Greek yoghurt or dairy-free yoghurt

- 1/4 cup of nuts or seeds (e.g., almonds or walnuts)

- Honey (optional, for drizzling)

Instructions:

For Assembling the Parfait:

1. Start by layering the bottom of a glass or a bowl with a portion of Greek yoghurt or dairy-free yoghurt.

2. Add a layer of fresh blueberries on top of the yoghurt.

3. Follow it with another layer of yoghurt.

4. Add a layer of fresh blackberries.

5. Continue to alternate layers of yoghurt and berries until the glass or bowl is filled.

6. Finish the parfait with a final layer of yoghurt on top.

For Garnishing:

1. Sprinkle the nuts or seeds (e.g., almonds or walnuts) on the top layer of yoghurt.

2. If desired, drizzle a touch of honey over the parfait for added sweetness. Keep in mind that honey is optional and can be omitted if you prefer a lower-sugar option.

Nutritional Information (approximate):

• Serving Size: 1 parfait (without honey)

• Calories: 300–350 kcal

• Protein: 15-20g

• Fat: 10-15g

• Carbohydrates: 35-40g

• Fibre: 10-12g

• Sugars: 15-20g

• Cholesterol: 10-15mg

• Sodium: 70-90mg

Strawberry Spinach Salad

Ingredients:

• 2 cups of fresh strawberries, hulled and sliced

• 4 cups of fresh spinach leaves

• 1/4 red onion, thinly sliced

• 1/2 cup of walnuts, chopped

• 1/4 cup of balsamic vinaigrette dressing

Instructions:

For preparing the salad:

1. Start by washing and drying the fresh strawberries and spinach leaves. Hull the strawberries and slice them into bite-sized pieces.

2. In a large salad bowl, combine the fresh spinach leaves, sliced strawberries, and thinly sliced red onion.

3. Toss the ingredients gently to distribute them evenly in the bowl.

For making the salad dressing:

1. In a separate small bowl, prepare the balsamic vinaigrette dressing. You can use a store-bought dressing or make your own by mixing balsamic vinegar and olive oil in a 1:3 ratio. If desired, add a touch of honey or sweetener to taste.

For Serving:

1. Drizzle the prepared balsamic vinaigrette dressing over the salad.

2. Sprinkle the chopped walnuts on top for added crunch and nutrition.

3. Toss the salad again to ensure that the dressing is evenly distributed.

Nutritional Information (approximate):

• Serving Size: 1 large salad serving (without homemade dressing)

• Calories: 200-250 kcal

• Protein: 4-6g

• Fat: 10-12g

• Carbohydrates: 25-30g

• Fibre: 6-8g

- Sugars: 14-16g
- Cholesterol: 0mg
- Sodium: 120-140mg

Plum and Cherry Smoothie

Ingredients:

- 2 ripe plums, pitted and sliced
- 1 cup of fresh or frozen cherries, pitted
- 1 cup of Greek yoghurt or dairy-free yoghurt
- Honey (optional, for added sweetness)
- Ice (optional, for a colder smoothie)

Instructions:

For preparing the smoothie:

1. Begin by washing and preparing the plums. Remove the pits and slice the plums into smaller pieces.

2. If you're using fresh cherries, make sure to pit them as well. If you prefer a colder smoothie, you can use frozen cherries.

3. In a blender, combine the sliced plums, cherries, and Greek yoghurt (or a dairy-free alternative).

4. If you desire added sweetness, you can include a drizzle of honey at this point. Start with a small amount and adjust to your preferred level of sweetness.

5. If you'd like a colder smoothie, add a handful of ice to the blender.

6. Blend the ingredients until you achieve a smooth and

creamy consistency. You can add a little water or more yoghurt if needed to reach your desired thickness.

7. Taste the smoothie and adjust the sweetness or consistency by adding more honey or yoghurt if necessary.

Nutritional Information (approximate):

• Serving Size: 1 smoothie (without honey)

• Calories: 200-250 kcal

• Protein: 8-10g

• Fat: 2-4g

• Carbohydrates: 40-45g

• Fibre: 6-8g

• Sugars: 30-35g

• Cholesterol: 10-15mg

• Sodium: 30-40mg

Blueberry Chicken Salad

Ingredients:

• 1 cup of fresh blueberries

• 2 grilled chicken breasts, sliced

• 4 cups of mixed greens (e.g., spinach, arugula, and romaine)

• 1/2 cup of almonds, sliced or slivered

• 1/4 cup of balsamic vinaigrette dressing

Instructions:

For grilling the chicken:

1. Season the chicken breasts with a touch of salt and freshly ground black pepper.

2. Preheat your grill to medium-high heat (about 400–450°F or 200–230°C).

3. Grill the chicken breasts for about 6–8 minutes on each side, or until they are fully cooked and have nice grill marks. The internal temperature of the chicken should reach 165°F (74°C).

4. Once done, remove the chicken from the grill and let it rest for a few minutes before slicing.

Assembling the Salad:

1. Start by washing and drying the mixed greens.

2. In a large salad bowl, combine the mixed greens, fresh blueberries, and sliced grilled chicken.

3. Toss the ingredients gently to distribute them evenly in the bowl.

For making the salad dressing:

1. In a small bowl, prepare the balsamic vinaigrette dressing. You can use a store-bought dressing or make your own by mixing balsamic vinegar and olive oil in a 1:3 ratio. You can also add a touch of honey or sweetener to taste.

For Serving:

1. Drizzle the prepared balsamic vinaigrette dressing over the salad.

2. Sprinkle the sliced or slivered almonds on top for added crunch and nutrition.

3. Toss the salad again to ensure that the dressing is evenly distributed.

Nutritional Information (approximate):

• Serving Size: 1 large salad serving (without homemade dressing)

• Calories: 350-400 kcal

• Protein: 30-35g

• Fat: 15-20g

• Carbohydrates: 20-25g

• Fibre: 5-7g

• Sugars: 10-12g

• Cholesterol: 80-100mg

• Sodium: 300-350mg

Blackberry Chia Pudding

Ingredients:

• 1 cup of fresh blackberries

• 3 tablespoons of chia seeds

• 1 cup of almond milk or coconut milk

• Honey (optional, for added sweetness)

Instructions:

For preparing the pudding:

1. Begin by washing and drying the fresh blackberries.

2. In a blender or food processor, blend the blackberries until you have a smooth puree. If desired, you can strain the puree to remove seeds, but they are also nutritious and can be kept if preferred.

3. In a bowl, combine the blackberry puree and chia seeds.

4. Mix well to ensure that the chia seeds are evenly distributed in the puree.

5. Pour in the almond milk or coconut milk and stir until all the ingredients are well combined.

6. If you desire added sweetness, you can include a drizzle of honey at this point. Start with a small amount and adjust to your preferred level of sweetness.

7. Cover the bowl and refrigerate the mixture for at least 2 hours or overnight to allow it to set. The chia seeds will absorb the liquid and create a pudding-like consistency.

Nutritional Information (approximate):

• Serving Size: 1 serving (without honey)

• Calories: 200-250 kcal

• Protein: 6-8g

• Fat: 8-10g

• Carbohydrates: 30-35g

• Fibre: 14-16g

• Sugars: 15-18g

• Cholesterol: 0mg

• Sodium: 30-40mg

CHAPTER 7

Vegetables:

Sauteed Spinach with Garlic and Olive Oil

Ingredients:

• 8 cups of fresh spinach leaves

• 4 cloves of garlic, minced

• 2 tablespoons of extra-virgin olive oil

• Salt and freshly ground black pepper, to taste

Instructions:

For preparing the spinach:

1. Begin by washing and drying the fresh spinach leaves. You can use a salad spinner or paper towels to remove excess moisture.

2. If the spinach leaves are large, you can chop or tear them into smaller pieces.

For Sauteing:

1. In a large skillet or pan, heat the extra-virgin olive oil over medium heat.

2. Add the minced garlic to the hot oil and sauté for about 30 seconds, or until it becomes fragrant. Be careful not to brown the garlic, as it can become bitter.

3. Carefully add the fresh spinach to the pan. Use tongs or a spatula to gently toss and stir the spinach.

4. Continue to sauté the spinach until it wilts and becomes tender, which should take about 2–3 minutes.

5. Season the sauteed spinach with a touch of salt and freshly ground black pepper. Be cautious with the salt, as spinach can be naturally salty.

6. Once the spinach is wilted and seasoned to your liking, remove the pan from the heat.

Nutritional Information (approximate):

• Serving Size: 1 cup of sauteed spinach

• Calories: 50–60 kcal

• Protein: 3-4g

• Fat: 4-5g

• Carbohydrates: 3-4g

• Fibre: 2-3g

• Sugars: 0-1g

• Cholesterol: 0mg

• Sodium: 50-60mg

Kale and Quinoa Salad with Lemon Vinaigrette

Ingredients:

For the salad:

• 4 cups of kale, stems removed, and leaves thinly sliced

• 1 cup of quinoa, cooked and cooled

• 1 cup of cherry tomatoes, halved

• 1/2 cup of red onion, thinly sliced

For the lemon vinaigrette:

• 3 tablespoons of freshly squeezed lemon juice

• 2 tablespoons of extra-virgin olive oil

• 1 teaspoon of Dijon mustard

• Salt and freshly ground black pepper, to taste

Instructions:

Preparing the Quinoa:

1. Begin by rinsing the quinoa in a fine-mesh strainer under cold running water. This helps remove the bitter outer coating.

2. In a saucepan, combine the rinsed quinoa with 2 cups of water. Bring to a boil.

3. Reduce the heat to low, cover the saucepan, and simmer for 15 minutes, or until the quinoa is cooked and the liquid is absorbed.

4. Remove the saucepan from the heat, let it sit for 5 minutes, and then fluff the quinoa with a fork.

5. Allow the quinoa to cool to room temperature.

For making the lemon vinaigrette:

1. In a small bowl, whisk together the freshly squeezed lemon juice, extra-virgin olive oil, Dijon mustard, salt, and freshly ground black pepper. Adjust the seasoning to your taste.

2. The lemon vinaigrette can be made ahead of time and stored in the refrigerator until you're ready to use it.

Assembling the Salad:

1. In a large salad bowl, combine the thinly sliced kale, cooked and cooled quinoa, halved cherry tomatoes, and thinly sliced red onion.

2. Drizzle the lemon vinaigrette over the salad.

3. Toss the salad gently to ensure that the dressing is evenly distributed.

4. Allow the salad to rest for a few minutes to allow the flavours to meld.

Nutritional Information (approximate):

• Serving Size: 1 large salad serving

• Calories: 350-400 kcal

• Protein: 10-12g

• Fat: 10-12g

• Carbohydrates: 55-60g

• Fibre: 8-10g

• Sugars: 4-6g

• Cholesterol: 0mg

• Sodium: 200-250mg

Broccoli and Almond Stir-Fry

Ingredients:

• 4 cups of broccoli florets

• 1/2 cup of slivered almonds

• 2 cloves of garlic, minced

• 2 tablespoons of soy sauce or tamari (for a gluten-free option)

• 2 tablespoons of sesame oil

Instructions:

For preparing the broccoli:

1. Start by washing and drying the broccoli florets. You can also purchase pre-cut florets for convenience.

2. If the florets are large, you can chop them into smaller, bite-sized pieces.

For making the stir-fry:

1. In a wok or a large skillet, heat the sesame oil over medium-high heat.

2. Add the minced garlic to the hot oil and sauté for about 30 seconds, or until it becomes fragrant.

3. Carefully add the broccoli florets to the pan. Use tongs or a spatula to stir-fry the broccoli. You can also add a few tablespoons of water to create some steam and help the broccoli cook more evenly.

4. Continue to stir-fry the broccoli for about 3–4 minutes,

or until it becomes bright green and tender but still slightly crisp.

5. Add the slivered almonds to the pan and continue to stir-fry for an additional 1-2 minutes. The almonds should become lightly toasted.

6. Drizzle the soy sauce or tamari over the stir-fry and toss the ingredients to coat them evenly. You can adjust the amount of soy sauce or tamari to suit your taste.

7. Once the broccoli is tender and the almonds are toasted, remove the pan from the heat.

Nutritional Information (approximate):

• Serving Size: 1 cup of stir-fry

• Calories: 150-200 kcal

• Protein: 6-8g

• Fat: 10-12g

• Carbohydrates: 10-12g

• Fibre: 4-6g

• Sugars: 2-3g

• Cholesterol: 0mg

• Sodium: 450-550mg

Brussels sprouts and bacon hash

Ingredients:

• 4 cups of Brussels sprouts, trimmed and halved

• 4 slices of bacon, chopped

- 1 medium onion, finely chopped
- 2 cloves of garlic, minced
- 2 tablespoons of olive oil
- Salt and freshly ground black pepper, to taste

Instructions:

For preparing the Brussels sprouts:

1. Start by trimming the stem ends of the Brussels sprouts, and then halve them.

2. Rinse the halved Brussels sprouts under cold, running water and pat them dry.

For Making the Hash:

1. In a large skillet or pan, heat the olive oil over medium-high heat.

2. Add the chopped bacon to the hot oil and sauté for about 3–4 minutes, or until it becomes crispy.

3. Using a slotted spoon, remove the crispy bacon from the pan and place it on a paper towel-lined plate to drain excess grease.

4. In the same skillet with the bacon drippings, add the finely chopped onion and minced garlic. Sauté for about 2–3 minutes, or until the onion becomes translucent.

5. Add the halved Brussels sprouts to the skillet. Stir-fry them for about 8–10 minutes, or until they are tender and slightly browned. Adjust the cooking time to achieve your preferred level of doneness.

6. Return the crispy bacon to the skillet and toss it with the Brussels sprouts.

7. Season the hash with salt and freshly ground black

pepper, to taste. Be cautious with the salt, as bacon is naturally salty.

8. Once the hash is cooked to your satisfaction, remove the pan from the heat.

Nutritional Information (approximate):

• Serving Size: 1 cup of Brussels sprouts and bacon hash

• Calories: 250–300 kcal

• Protein: 10-12g

• Fat: 20-22g

• Carbohydrates: 10-12g

• Fibre: 4-6g

• Sugars: 2-3g

• Cholesterol: 25-30mg

• Sodium: 350-400mg

Collard greens with smoked turkey

Ingredients:

• 1 bunch of collard greens, stems removed, and leaves chopped

• 1 smoked turkey leg (or smoked turkey wings or neck)

• 1 medium onion, finely chopped

• 3 cloves of garlic, minced

• 4 cups of low-sodium chicken broth

• Red pepper flakes (optional, for added heat)

• Salt and freshly ground black pepper, to taste

Instructions:

For preparing the collar greens:

1. Start by washing and drying the collard greens. Remove the tough stems by slicing along each side of the stem and then chopping the leaves into bite-sized pieces.

2. Rinse the chopped collard greens under cold, running water.

For cooking the smoked turkey:

1. In a large pot, place the smoked turkey leg (or other smoked turkey parts) and add enough water to cover it.

2. Bring the water to a boil, then reduce the heat to low, cover, and simmer for 45–60 minutes, or until the turkey is fully cooked and tender. The exact cooking time may vary based on the size of the turkey leg or parts.

3. Once cooked, remove the smoked turkey from the pot, let it cool, and then shred the meat into smaller pieces.

For Making the Collard Greens:

1. In a large pot, heat a small amount of olive oil or use a non-stick cooking spray over medium heat.

2. Add the chopped onion and minced garlic to the pot and sauté for about 2-3 minutes, or until they become fragrant and the onion is translucent.

3. Add the chopped collard greens to the pot. Stir them well with the sautéed onion and garlic.

4. Pour in the low-sodium chicken broth to cover the collard greens.

5. If you prefer some heat, add red pepper flakes at this point.

6. Bring the liquid to a simmer, then reduce the heat to low, cover the pot, and cook for about 45–60 minutes, or until the collard greens are tender. Stir occasionally.

7. When the collard greens are tender, add the shredded smoked turkey to the pot and stir it into the greens.

8. Season with salt and freshly ground black pepper, to taste. Be cautious with the salt, as the smoked turkey can be salty.

9. Allow the flavours to meld by letting the collard greens and smoked turkey simmer together for an additional 10–15 minutes.

Nutritional Information (approximate):

• Serving Size: 1 cup of collard greens with smoked turkey

• Calories: 150-200 kcal

• Protein: 12-15g

• Fat: 4-6g

• Carbohydrates: 15-18g

• Fibre: 5-7g

• Sugars: 3-5g

• Cholesterol: 35-40mg

• Sodium: 600-700mg

CHAPTER 8

Healthy Fats:

Mediterranean Salad with Olive Oil Dressing

Ingredients:

For the salad:

• 4 cups of mixed greens

• 1 cup of cherry tomatoes, halved

• 1 cucumber, thinly sliced

• 1/2 red onion, thinly sliced

• 1/2 cup of Kalamata olives, pitted

For the olive oil dressing:

• 3 tablespoons of extra virgin olive oil

• 2 tablespoons of freshly squeezed lemon juice

• 1 tablespoon of fresh oregano, finely chopped

• Salt and freshly ground black pepper, to taste

Instructions:

For making the salad:

1. Begin by washing and drying the mixed greens. You can use a salad spinner or paper towels to remove excess

moisture.

2. In a large salad bowl, combine the mixed greens, halved cherry tomatoes, thinly sliced cucumber, thinly sliced red onion, and pitted Kalamata olives. Toss the ingredients gently to distribute them evenly.

For making the olive oil dressing:

1. In a small bowl, whisk together the extra virgin olive oil, freshly squeezed lemon juice, finely chopped fresh oregano, salt, and freshly ground black pepper. Adjust the seasoning to your taste.

2. The olive oil dressing can be made ahead of time and stored in the refrigerator until you're ready to use it.

For Dressing the Salad:

1. Drizzle the olive oil dressing over the salad. Toss the salad gently to ensure that the dressing is evenly distributed.

2. Allow the salad to rest for a few minutes to let the flavours meld.

Nutritional Information (approximate):

• Serving Size: 1 large salad serving

• Calories: 150-200 kcal

• Protein: 2-3g

• Fat: 12-15g

• Carbohydrates: 12-15g

• Fibre: 3-4g

• Sugars: 5-6g

• Cholesterol: 0mg

• Sodium: 200-250mg

Grilled Chicken with Lemon and Olive Oil Marinade

Ingredients:

• 4 boneless, skinless chicken breasts or thighs

• 1/4 cup extra virgin olive oil

• 1/4 cup fresh lemon juice

• 3 cloves of garlic, minced

• 2 tablespoons of fresh rosemary, finely chopped

• Salt and freshly ground black pepper, to taste

Instructions:

For making the marinade:

1. In a bowl, combine the extra virgin olive oil, fresh lemon juice, minced garlic, finely chopped fresh rosemary, salt, and freshly ground black pepper. Whisk the ingredients together to create the marinade.

2. Reserve a small portion of the marinade (about 2-3 tablespoons) for basting during grilling.

For Marinating the Chicken:

1. Place the chicken breasts or thighs in a resealable plastic bag or a shallow dish.

2. Pour the marinade over the chicken, making sure each piece is well coated. Seal the bag or cover the dish, and refrigerate for at least 30 minutes. You can marinate the chicken for up to 4 hours for maximum flavour.

For grilling the chicken:

1. Preheat your grill to medium-high heat (about 375–

400°F or 190–205°C).

2. Remove the chicken from the marinade and discard the used marinade.

3. Grill the chicken for about 6-7 minutes per side for chicken breasts or 8-10 minutes per side for chicken thighs. The internal temperature of the chicken should reach 165°F (74°C), and the juices should run clear.

4. During the last few minutes of grilling, use the reserved marinade to baste the chicken for added flavour.

5. Once the chicken is cooked through and has grill marks, remove it from the grill.

Nutritional Information (approximate):

• Serving Size: 1 chicken breast or thigh

• Calories: 200-250 kcal

• Protein: 25-30g

• Fat: 10-12g

• Carbohydrates: 2-3g

• Fibre: 0g

• Sugars: 0g

• Cholesterol: 70-80mg

• Sodium: 50-60mg

Flaxseed and Berry Smoothies

Ingredients:

• 1 tablespoon of flaxseed oil

• 1 cup of mixed berries (e.g., blueberries, strawberries,

raspberries)

- 1/2 cup of Greek yoghurt or dairy-free yoghurt

- 1-2 teaspoons of honey (optional, for sweetness)

- 1/2 cup of ice

Instructions:

For making the smoothie:

1. In a blender, add the flaxseed oil, mixed berries, Greek yoghurt (or dairy-free alternative), and ice.

2. If you prefer your smoothie to be on the sweeter side, you can add honey to taste. Start with 1 teaspoon, blend, and then adjust as needed.

3. Blend all the ingredients on high until the mixture is smooth and has a creamy consistency.

4. If the smoothie is too thick, you can add a little more yoghurt or a splash of water to reach your preferred consistency.

Nutritional Information (approximate):

- Serving size: 1 smoothie

- Calories: 250–300 kcal

- Protein: 8-10g

- Fat: 16-18g

- Carbohydrates: 20-25g

- Fibre: 5-7g

- Sugars: 15-18g

- Cholesterol: 10-15mg

- Sodium: 50-60mg

Roasted Vegetables with Olive Oil and Herbs

Ingredients:

• Assorted vegetables (e.g., bell peppers, zucchini, eggplant, cherry tomatoes)

• 2-3 tablespoons of extra virgin olive oil

• 3 cloves of garlic, minced

• Fresh herbs (e.g., thyme, basil, rosemary), finely chopped

• Salt and freshly ground black pepper, to taste

Instructions:

For preparing the vegetables:

1. Preheat your oven to 425°F (220°C).

2. Wash, peel (if necessary), and chop the assorted vegetables into bite-sized pieces. You can use a variety of vegetables, like bell peppers, zucchini, eggplant, and cherry tomatoes.

3. If you're using cherry tomatoes, it's best to keep them whole.

For seasoning and roasting:

1. In a large mixing bowl, combine the chopped vegetables, extra virgin olive oil, minced garlic, and the finely chopped fresh herbs. Toss the ingredients together to coat the vegetables evenly with the oil and herbs.

2. Season the vegetables with salt and freshly ground black pepper, to taste. Adjust the seasoning to your preference.

For Roasting:

1. Spread the seasoned vegetables in a single layer on a

baking sheet or a roasting pan. Make sure they are not overcrowded to allow even roasting.

2. Place the baking sheet or roasting pan in the preheated oven and roast for about 20–25 minutes, or until the vegetables are tender and have developed a slight caramelization.

3. About halfway through the roasting time, you can flip or stir the vegetables for even cooking.

Nutritional Information (approximate):

• Serving Size: 1 cup of roasted vegetables

• Calories: 80-100 kcal

• Protein: 2-3g

• Fat: 7-9g

• Carbohydrates: 5-7g

• Fibre: 2-3g

• Sugars: 3-4g

• Cholesterol: 0mg

• Sodium: 30-40mg

Avocado and Tomato Bruschetta

Ingredients:

• 1 ripe avocado, peeled, pitted, and diced

• 2 ripe tomatoes, diced

• 1/4 cup of fresh basil leaves, thinly sliced

• 2 tablespoons of extra virgin olive oil

• 1 tablespoon of balsamic vinegar

• 1 whole-grain or gluten-free baguette, sliced into 1/2-inch-thick pieces

Instructions:

Preparing the Bruschetta:

1. In a large mixing bowl, combine the diced avocado, diced tomatoes, and thinly sliced fresh basil.

2. Drizzle the extra virgin olive oil and balsamic vinegar over the avocado, tomatoes, and basil.

3. Gently toss the ingredients to ensure they are well coated with the olive oil and balsamic vinegar.

For toasting the baguette:

1. Preheat your oven's broiler or grill to high heat.

2. Place the baguette slices on a baking sheet or grill grates.

3. Toast the baguette slices for about 1-2 minutes on each side or until they become golden brown and slightly crispy.

Assembling the Bruschetta:

1. Spoon the avocado and tomato mixture onto each toasted baguette slice.

2. Garnish with additional fresh basil leaves, if desired.

Nutritional Information (approximate):

• Serving Size: 2 bruschetta slices

• Calories: 200-250 kcal

• Protein: 4-6g

• Fat: 12-15g

• Carbohydrates: 20-25g

• Fibre: 4-5g

• Sugars: 2-4g

• Cholesterol: 0mg

• Sodium: 150-200mg

CHAPTER 9

Nuts and Seeds:

Walnut-Crusted Salmon

Ingredients:

• 4 salmon fillets (6–8 ounces each)

• 1/2 cup chopped walnuts

• 2 tablespoons Dijon mustard

• 1 tablespoon of fresh lemon juice

• 2 tablespoons fresh dill, finely chopped

• Salt and freshly ground black pepper, to taste

Instructions:

For Preparing the Walnut-Crusted Salmon:

1. Preheat your oven to 400°F (200°C).

2. Place the chopped walnuts, Dijon mustard, fresh lemon juice, and finely chopped fresh dill in a bowl. Mix the ingredients together to form a crumbly paste.

3. Season the salmon fillets with a pinch of salt and freshly ground black pepper.

4. Spread the walnut mixture evenly over the top of each salmon fillet, pressing it gently to adhere.

For baking the salmon:

1. Place the salmon fillets on a baking sheet lined with parchment paper or lightly greased.

2. Bake the salmon in the preheated oven for approximately 12–15 minutes, or until the salmon flakes easily with a fork and the walnut crust is golden brown.

3. If you prefer a more well-done salmon, you can bake it for an additional 3–5 minutes.

Nutritional Information (approximate):

• Serving Size: 1 salmon fillet

• Calories: 350-400 kcal

• Protein: 35-40g

• Fat: 20-25g

• Carbohydrates: 5-7g

• Fibre: 2-3g

• Sugars: 1-2g

• Cholesterol: 90-100mg

• Sodium: 250-300mg

Flaxseed and Berry Smoothies

Ingredients:

• 1 tablespoon of flaxseeds

• 1 cup of mixed berries (e.g., blueberries, strawberries, raspberries)

• 1/2 cup of Greek yoghurt or dairy-free yoghurt

• 1-2 teaspoons of honey (optional, for sweetness)

• 1/2 cup of ice

Instructions:

For making the smoothie:

1. In a blender, add the flaxseeds, mixed berries, Greek yoghurt (or dairy-free alternative), and ice.

2. If you prefer your smoothie to be on the sweeter side, you can add honey to taste. Start with 1 teaspoon, blend, and then adjust as needed.

3. Blend all the ingredients on high until the mixture is smooth and has a creamy consistency.

4. If the smoothie is too thick, you can add a little more yoghurt or a splash of water to reach your preferred consistency.

Nutritional Information (approximate):

• Serving size: 1 smoothie

• Calories: 200-250 kcal

• Protein: 8-10g

• Fat: 16-18g

• Carbohydrates: 20-25g

• Fibre: 5-7g

• Sugars: 15-18g

• Cholesterol: 10-15mg

• Sodium: 50-60mg

Almond-encrusted chicken tenders

Ingredients:

- 1 pound of chicken tenders
- 1 cup ground almonds
- 1 teaspoon paprika
- 1/2 teaspoon garlic powder
- 2-3 tablespoons olive oil
- Salt and freshly ground black pepper, to taste

Instructions:

For preparing the chicken tenders:

1. Preheat your oven to 400°F (200°C).

2. In a shallow dish, combine the ground almonds, paprika, garlic powder, salt, and freshly ground black pepper.

3. Pat the chicken tenders dry with paper towels. This helps the almond mixture stick better to the chicken.

For coating the chicken tenders:

1. One at a time, dip each chicken tender into the olive oil, ensuring it's well coated.

2. Next, press the oiled chicken tender into the almond mixture, coating it evenly with the almond mixture. Press the almond mixture onto the chicken to make it stick.

For baking the chicken tenders:

1. Place the coated chicken tenders on a baking sheet lined with parchment paper or a greased oven-safe rack.

2. Bake in the preheated oven for about 15-20 minutes or until the chicken is cooked through and the almond coating is golden brown and crispy.

3. Serve the almond-encrusted chicken tenders hot with your favourite dipping sauce.

Nutritional Information (approximate):

• Serving Size: 3-4 chicken tenders

• Calories: 350-400 kcal

• Protein: 25-30g

• Fat: 25-30g

• Carbohydrates: 6-8g

• Fibre: 3-4g

• Sugars: 1-2g

• Cholesterol: 75-90mg

• Sodium: 350-400mg

Spinach and Walnut Salad

Ingredients:

• 6 cups of fresh spinach leaves

• 1/2 cup chopped walnuts

• 1/4 cup finely chopped red onion

• 1/4 cup crumbled feta cheese (in moderation)

• 2-3 tablespoons balsamic vinaigrette dressing

Instructions:

For preparing the salad:

1. In a large salad bowl, place the fresh spinach leaves.

2. Sprinkle the chopped walnuts evenly over the spinach.

3. Add the finely chopped red onion to the salad.

4. Crumble the feta cheese in moderation and sprinkle it over the salad.

For Dressing the Salad:

1. Drizzle 2-3 tablespoons of balsamic vinaigrette dressing over the salad. Start with a smaller amount and add more according to your taste preference.

2. Gently toss the salad to ensure all the ingredients are coated with the dressing.

3. Serve the spinach and walnut salad immediately as a side dish or a light meal.

Nutritional Information (approximate):

• Serving Size: 1.5 cups of salad

• Calories: 250–300 kcal

• Protein: 8-10g

• Fat: 18-20g

• Carbohydrates: 14-16g

• Fibre: 4-5g

• Sugars: 4-6g

• Cholesterol: 15-20mg

• Sodium: 350-400mg

Flaxseed Porridge with Berries

Ingredients:

• 2 tablespoons of flaxseeds

• 1/2 cup of rolled oats (gluten-free, if preferred)

• 1/2 cup of mixed berries (e.g., blueberries, strawberries, raspberries)

• 1/2 cup of Greek yoghurt or dairy-free yoghurt

• 1-2 teaspoons of honey (optional, for sweetness)

Instructions:

For preparing the porridge:

1. In a small saucepan, combine the flaxseeds and rolled oats with 1 cup of water. Bring to a gentle simmer.

2. Stir the mixture and let it cook over low to medium heat for about 5-7 minutes, or until it thickens to your desired consistency.

3. Remove the porridge from the heat and let it cool slightly.

For serving the porridge:

1. In a serving bowl, spoon the flaxseed porridge.

2. Top the porridge with mixed berries, placing them evenly over the surface.

3. Add a dollop of Greek yoghurt (or a dairy-free alternative) on top of the berries.

4. If you prefer a touch of sweetness, you can drizzle 1-2 teaspoons of honey over the yoghurt.

5. Serve the flaxseed porridge with berries warm and enjoy.

Nutritional Information (approximate):

• Serving Size: 1 bowl of porridge

• Calories: 300–350 kcal

• Protein: 10-12g

• Fat: 12-14g

• Carbohydrates: 40-45g

• Fibre: 8-10g

• Sugars: 10-12g

- Cholesterol: 5-10mg
- Sodium: 50-60mg

CHAPTER 10

Herbs and Spices:

Garlic and Herb Grilled Shrimp

Ingredients:

• 1 pound of large shrimp, peeled and deveined

• 3-4 cloves of garlic, minced

• 2-3 tablespoons of fresh herbs (e.g., rosemary, thyme, parsley), finely chopped

• Juice of 1 lemon

• 2-3 tablespoons of olive oil

• Salt and freshly ground black pepper, to taste

Instructions:

For Marinating the Shrimp:

1. In a bowl, combine the minced garlic, chopped fresh herbs, lemon juice, and olive oil. Mix well to create the marinade.

2. Season the peeled and deveined shrimp with a pinch of salt and freshly ground black pepper.

3. Place the shrimp in a resealable plastic bag or a shallow dish.

4. Pour the marinade over the shrimp and ensure that the

shrimp are well-coated. Seal the bag or cover the dish and refrigerate for 20-30 minutes.

For Grilling the Shrimp:

5. Preheat your grill to medium-high heat (about 400°F or 200°C).

6. Thread the marinated shrimp onto skewers, making sure not to overcrowd them.

7. Grill the shrimp for about 2-3 minutes per side or until they turn pink and opaque. Avoid overcooking, as shrimp cook quickly.

8. Once grilled, remove the shrimp from the skewers.

9. Serve the garlic and herb grilled shrimp hot with your favorite side dishes or a fresh salad.

Nutritional Information (Approximate):

• Serving Size: 4-5 grilled shrimp

• Calories: 100-120 kcal

• Protein: 20-24g

• Fat: 3-4g

• Carbohydrates: 2-3g

• Fiber: 0g

• Sugars: 0g

• Cholesterol: 150-200mg

• Sodium: 150-200mg

Ginger and Turmeric Chicken Stir-Fry

Ingredients:

- 1 pound of boneless, skinless chicken breast, cut into thin strips
- 1 tablespoon of fresh ginger, minced
- 1 teaspoon of ground turmeric
- 2 bell peppers (red, yellow, or green), thinly sliced
- 2 cups of broccoli florets
- 2-3 tablespoons of low-sodium soy sauce or tamari
- 1-2 tablespoons of olive oil or sesame oil
- Salt and freshly ground black pepper, to taste

Instructions:

For Preparing the Stir-Fry:

1. In a bowl, combine the chicken strips with minced ginger and ground turmeric. Allow the chicken to marinate for about 10-15 minutes.

2. Heat a wok or large skillet over medium-high heat and add 1-2 tablespoons of olive oil or sesame oil.

3. Add the marinated chicken strips to the hot wok or skillet. Stir-fry for about 5-7 minutes or until the chicken is cooked through and turns golden brown. Remove the cooked chicken from the wok and set it aside.

4. In the same wok or skillet, add a little more oil if needed and add the bell peppers and broccoli. Stir-fry for about 3-4 minutes until the vegetables become tender but still crisp.

5. Return the cooked chicken to the wok with the vegetables.

6. Drizzle low-sodium soy sauce or tamari over the mixture and toss everything together.

7. Continue to stir-fry for another 2-3 minutes until all the

ingredients are well combined and heated through.

8. Season with salt and freshly ground black pepper to taste.

9. Serve the ginger and turmeric chicken stir-fry hot, as it is or over a bed of cooked quinoa or brown rice.

Nutritional Information (Approximate):

• Serving Size: 1/4 of the recipe (without rice or quinoa)

• Calories: 250-300 kcal

• Protein: 25-30g

• Fat: 10-12g

• Carbohydrates: 10-12g

• Fiber: 3-4g

• Sugars: 4-5g

• Cholesterol: 70-80mg

• Sodium: 400-450mg

Parsley and Lemon Quinoa Salad

Ingredients:

• 1 cup of quinoa

• 1/2 cup of fresh parsley, finely chopped

• Zest and juice of 1 lemon

• 1 cup of cherry tomatoes, halved

• 1 cucumber, diced

• Salt and freshly ground black pepper, to taste

• Olive oil (optional)

Instructions:

For Cooking the Quinoa:

1. Rinse the quinoa under cold water in a fine-mesh sieve to remove any bitterness.

2. In a medium saucepan, combine the rinsed quinoa with 2 cups of water. Bring to a boil.

3. Reduce the heat to low, cover, and let it simmer for about 15 minutes or until the quinoa is cooked and the water is absorbed.

4. Remove the saucepan from the heat and let it sit for 5 minutes, covered. Then, fluff the quinoa with a fork and let it cool.

For Assembling the Salad:

5. In a large mixing bowl, combine the cooked and cooled quinoa, chopped fresh parsley, lemon zest, lemon juice, halved cherry tomatoes, and diced cucumber.

6. Gently toss all the ingredients until they are well mixed.

7. Season with salt and freshly ground black pepper to taste. If you prefer, you can drizzle a bit of olive oil for added flavor.

8. Refrigerate the parsley and lemon quinoa salad for at least 30 minutes before serving to let the flavors meld.

9. Serve the salad cold as a refreshing and nutritious side dish or as a light main course.

Nutritional Information (Approximate):

• Serving Size: 1/4 of the recipe (about 1.5 cups)

• Calories: 180-200 kcal

• Protein: 6-8g

• Fat: 4-6g

• Carbohydrates: 30-35g

• Fiber: 4-5g

• Sugars: 3-4g

• Cholesterol: 0mg

• Sodium: 10-15mg

Rosemary and Garlic Roasted Potatoes

Ingredients:

• 1 pound of baby potatoes, washed and halved

• 2-3 sprigs of fresh rosemary, leaves removed and finely chopped

• 3-4 cloves of garlic, minced

• 2-3 tablespoons of olive oil

• Salt and freshly ground black pepper, to taste

Instructions:

1. Preheat the Oven: Preheat your oven to 425°F (220°C). This high temperature will help create crispy, delicious roasted potatoes.

2. Prepare the Potatoes: Wash the baby potatoes thoroughly, and if they are large, cut them in halves to ensure even cooking.

3. Prepare the Seasoning: In a small bowl, combine the minced garlic, finely chopped rosemary leaves, and olive oil. Mix well to create a fragrant herb-infused oil.

4. Toss and Season: Place the halved baby potatoes in a large mixing bowl. Drizzle the herb-infused oil over the potatoes. Season with salt and freshly ground black pepper to taste.

5. Coat and Mix: Toss the potatoes in the herb-infused oil until they are evenly coated. Make sure the garlic and rosemary are spread out evenly over the potatoes.

6. Arrange on a Baking Sheet: Line a baking sheet with parchment paper or lightly grease it. Spread the seasoned baby potatoes in a single layer on the baking sheet. This will ensure that they roast evenly and become crispy.

7. Roast the Potatoes: Place the baking sheet in the preheated oven and roast for about 25-30 minutes or until the potatoes are tender and golden brown. You can check for doneness by inserting a fork or knife into a potato – it should go in easily.

8. Serve: Once the potatoes are done, remove them from the oven and let them cool for a couple of minutes. Serve the rosemary and garlic roasted potatoes as a delicious and fragrant side dish.

Nutritional Information (Approximate):

• Serving Size: 1/4 of the recipe

• Calories: 150-180 kcal

• Protein: 2-3g

• Fat: 7-9g

• Carbohydrates: 20-25g

• Fiber: 2-3g

• Sugars: 1-2g

• Cholesterol: 0mg

• Sodium: 200-250mg

Herb-Marinated Grilled Lamb

Ingredients:

• 4 lamb chops or a leg of lamb (approx. 1.5 lbs or 680g)

• 4 cloves of garlic, minced

• 2-3 tablespoons of fresh herbs (e.g., mint, oregano), finely chopped

• Juice of 1 lemon

• 3-4 tablespoons of extra virgin olive oil

• Salt and freshly ground black pepper, to taste

Instructions:

1. Prepare the Marinade: In a bowl, combine the minced garlic, finely chopped fresh herbs, lemon juice, extra virgin olive oil, salt, and freshly ground black pepper. Mix well to create a fragrant herb-infused marinade.

2. Marinate the Lamb: Place the lamb chops or leg of lamb in a large, shallow dish. Pour the herb marinade over the lamb, making sure it's evenly coated. Massage the marinade into the lamb to ensure the flavors penetrate the meat. Cover the dish with plastic wrap and refrigerate for at least 2-4 hours, or ideally overnight for maximum flavor.

3. Prepare the Grill: Preheat your grill to medium-high heat (about 400-450°F or 200-230°C). Ensure the grates are clean and lightly oiled to prevent sticking.

4. Grill the Lamb: Remove the lamb from the refrigerator and let it come to room temperature for about 30 minutes. This allows for more even cooking. Grill the lamb chops

or leg of lamb for approximately 3-4 minutes per side for medium-rare (adjust the time to your preferred level of doneness). For a leg of lamb, grill for approximately 15-20 minutes per side, depending on its thickness and your desired doneness.

5. Rest and Slice: Once the lamb is grilled to your liking, remove it from the grill and let it rest for a few minutes. This allows the juices to redistribute, ensuring a moist and flavorful result. Slice the leg of lamb or serve the lamb chops as desired.

6. Serve: Plate the herb-marinated grilled lamb and garnish with additional fresh herbs, if desired. Enjoy with your choice of side dishes or salads.

Nutritional Information (Approximate - for 4 lamb chops):

• Serving Size: 1 lamb chop (about 4 oz or 115g)

• Calories: 250-300 kcal

• Protein: 24-30g

• Fat: 16-20g

• Carbohydrates: 2-4g

• Fiber: 0g

• Sugars: 0g

• Cholesterol: 90-110mg

• Sodium: 60-70mg

CHAPTER 11

Green Tea with Lemon and Honey

Ingredients:

• 2 green tea bags or 2 teaspoons of loose-leaf green tea

• 4 cups of water

• Fresh lemon slices

• Honey (optional, to taste)

Instructions:

1. Boil the Water: Bring 4 cups of water to a boil in a kettle or a saucepan. Remove it from heat just before it reaches a rolling boil.

2. Warm the Teapot: While the water is heating, warm a teapot or teacup by rinsing it with hot tap water. This helps maintain the water temperature and ensures the tea brews evenly.

3. Add Green Tea: Place the green tea bags or loose-leaf green tea into the warmed teapot.

4. Pour Hot Water: Once the water is at the right temperature (about 175°F or 80°C), pour it over the tea bags or loose tea in the teapot.

5. Steep the Tea: Cover the teapot and let the green tea steep for 2-3 minutes. If you prefer a stronger tea, you can steep for up to 5 minutes, but be cautious not to oversteep, as green tea can become bitter.

6. Serve: Pour the green tea into your teacup. Add a slice of fresh lemon for a refreshing twist and a drizzle of honey if you desire a touch of sweetness.

7. Enjoy: Sip your green tea slowly, savoring the flavors and the soothing qualities. The lemon and honey can be adjusted to your taste preference.

Nutritional Information (Approximate - without honey):

• Serving Size: 1 cup (8 oz or 240ml)

• Calories: 0 kcal (may vary slightly based on the honey added)

• Protein: 0g

• Fat: 0g

• Carbohydrates: 0g

• Fiber: 0g

• Sugars: 0g

• Cholesterol: 0mg

• Sodium: 0mg

Chamomile and Lavender Herbal Tea

Ingredients:

• 2 chamomile tea bags or 2 teaspoons of loose-leaf chamomile

• 1 teaspoon dried lavender buds (optional)

• Honey (optional, to taste)

Instructions:

1. Boil Water: Bring 2 cups of water to a boil in a kettle or saucepan.

2. Warm the Teapot: While the water is heating, warm a teapot or teacup by rinsing it with hot tap water. This helps maintain the water temperature and ensures the tea brews evenly.

3. Add Chamomile and Lavender: Place the chamomile tea bags or loose-leaf chamomile and dried lavender buds into the warmed teapot.

4. Pour Hot Water: Once the water is at the right temperature (about 212°F or 100°C for chamomile tea), pour it over the tea and lavender in the teapot.

5. Steep the Tea: Cover the teapot and let the tea steep for about 5 minutes. Steeping time may be adjusted to suit your desired strength and flavor.

6. Serve: Pour the chamomile and lavender tea into your teacup. Add a drizzle of honey if you desire a touch of sweetness.

7. Enjoy: Sip your chamomile and lavender herbal tea slowly, savoring the gentle and soothing flavors. The honey can be adjusted to your taste preference.

Nutritional Information (Approximate - without honey):

• Serving Size: 1 cup (8 oz or 240ml)

• Calories: 0 kcal (may vary slightly based on the honey

added)

- Protein: 0g

- Fat: 0g

- Carbohydrates: 0g

- Fiber: 0g

- Sugars: 0g

- Cholesterol: 0mg

- Sodium: 0mg

Peppermint Infusion

Ingredients:

- 2 peppermint tea bags or 2 teaspoons of loose-leaf peppermint

- A few fresh mint leaves (optional)

- Honey (optional, to taste)

Instructions:

1. Boil Water: Bring 2 cups of water to a boil in a kettle or saucepan.

2. Warm the Teapot: While the water is heating, warm a teapot or teacup by rinsing it with hot tap water. This helps maintain the water temperature and ensures the tea brews evenly.

3. Add Peppermint: Place the peppermint tea bags or loose-leaf peppermint and a few fresh mint leaves into the warmed teapot.

4. Pour Hot Water: Once the water is at the right temperature (about 212°F or 100°C for peppermint tea),

pour it over the tea and mint in the teapot.

5. Steep the Tea: Cover the teapot and let the peppermint tea steep for about 5-7 minutes. Adjust the steeping time according to your taste preference.

6. Serve: Pour the peppermint infusion into your teacup. Add a drizzle of honey if you desire some sweetness.

7. Enjoy: Sip your peppermint infusion slowly, enjoying the refreshing and soothing qualities. The honey can be adjusted to your taste preference.

Nutritional Information (Approximate - without honey):

• Serving Size: 1 cup (8 oz or 240ml)

• Calories: 0 kcal (may vary slightly based on the honey added)

• Protein: 0g

• Fat: 0g

• Carbohydrates: 0g

• Fiber: 0g

• Sugars: 0g

• Cholesterol: 0mg

• Sodium: 0mg

Ginger and Lemon Green Tea

Ingredients:

• 2 green tea bags or 2 teaspoons of loose-leaf green tea

• 2-3 thin slices of fresh ginger

• 2-3 thin slices of fresh lemon

• Honey (optional, to taste)

Instructions:

1. Boil Water: Bring 2 cups of water to a boil in a kettle or saucepan.

2. Warm the Teapot: While the water is heating, warm a teapot or teacup by rinsing it with hot tap water. This helps maintain the water temperature and ensures the tea brews evenly.

3. Add Green Tea: Place the green tea bags or loose-leaf green tea into the warmed teapot.

4. Add Ginger and Lemon: Add the thin slices of fresh ginger and lemon to the teapot with the green tea.

5. Pour Hot Water: Once the water is at the right temperature (about 175°F or 80°C for green tea), pour it over the tea, ginger, and lemon in the teapot.

6. Steep the Tea: Cover the teapot and let the green tea steep for about 3-4 minutes. Adjust the steeping time to achieve your desired strength.

7. Serve: Pour the ginger and lemon green tea into your teacup. Add a drizzle of honey if you desire some sweetness.

8. Enjoy: Sip your ginger and lemon green tea slowly, appreciating the refreshing and invigorating flavors. The honey can be customized to your taste preference.

Nutritional Information (Approximate - without honey):

• Serving Size: 1 cup (8 oz or 240ml)

• Calories: 0 kcal (may vary slightly based on the honey added)

- Protein: 0g

- Fat: 0g

- Carbohydrates: 0g

- Fiber: 0g

- Sugars: 0g

- Cholesterol: 0mg

- Sodium: 0mg

Hibiscus and Berry Iced Tea

Ingredients:

- 2 hibiscus tea bags or 2 teaspoons of loose-leaf hibiscus tea

- 1 cup mixed berries (e.g., strawberries, blueberries)

- 4-5 fresh mint leaves

- Honey (optional, to taste)

- Ice cubes

Instructions:

1. Boil Water: Bring 2 cups of water to a boil in a kettle or saucepan.

2. Warm the Teapot: While the water is heating, warm a teapot or a heatproof pitcher by rinsing it with hot tap water. This helps maintain the water temperature and ensures the tea brews evenly.

3. Add Hibiscus Tea: Place the hibiscus tea bags or loose-leaf hibiscus tea into the warmed teapot or pitcher.

4. Add Boiling Water: Once the water is boiling, pour it over

the hibiscus tea in the teapot or pitcher.

5. Steep the Tea: Cover the teapot or pitcher and let the hibiscus tea steep for about 5-7 minutes. Adjust the steeping time to achieve your desired strength.

6. Muddle Berries and Mint: In a separate bowl or glass, lightly muddle the mixed berries and fresh mint leaves to release their flavors.

7. Add Berry-Mint Mixture: Add the muddled berry and mint mixture to the brewed hibiscus tea.

8. Cool and Sweeten: Allow the tea to cool to room temperature, then refrigerate it for at least 1-2 hours until it's cold. You can sweeten the tea with honey, if desired.

9. Serve: Fill a glass with ice cubes and pour the hibiscus and berry iced tea over the ice.

10. Enjoy: Garnish with extra berries, mint leaves, or a lemon slice, and enjoy your refreshing hibiscus and berry iced tea.

Nutritional Information (Approximate - without honey):

• Serving Size: 1 glass (8 oz or 240ml)

• Calories: 5-10 kcal (may vary slightly based on the honey added)

• Protein: 0g

• Fat: 0g

• Carbohydrates: 1-2g

• Fiber: 0-1g

• Sugars: 0-1g

• Cholesterol: 0mg

• Sodium: 0mg

CHAPTER 12

Meal Planning and Recipes

Here's a 14-day meal plan for a Blood Type O individual that includes a variety of breakfast, lunch, dinner, and snack options. This plan adheres to the general principles of the Blood Type O Diet, emphasizing lean meats, fish, poultry, specific fruits and vegetables, and limited grains and dairy.

Day 1:

Breakfast:

• Scrambled eggs with spinach and a side of fresh strawberries

Lunch:

• Grilled chicken salad with mixed greens, cherry tomatoes, and olive oil dressing

Dinner:

• Baked salmon with asparagus and a lemon-dill sauce

Snack:

• Celery sticks with almond butter

Day 2:

Breakfast:

• Greek yogurt with fresh blueberries and a drizzle of honey

Lunch:

• Turkey and avocado wrap with lettuce, tomato, and gluten-free tortilla

Dinner:

• Stir-fried lean beef with broccoli and ginger, served over cauliflower rice

Snack:

• Sliced apples with a sprinkle of cinnamon

Day 3:

Breakfast:

• Omelette with mushrooms, red bell peppers, and a side of sliced plums

Lunch:

• Spinach and kale salad with grilled shrimp, red onion, and vinaigrette

Dinner:

• Roasted chicken thighs with Brussels sprouts and olive oil

Snack:

• Carrot and cucumber sticks with hummus

Day 4:

Breakfast:

• Smoothie with almond milk, flaxseeds, mixed berries, and a scoop of protein powder

Lunch:

• Tuna salad with mixed greens, celery, and olive oil dressing

Dinner:

• Grilled lamb chops with a mint and garlic marinade, served with steamed green beans

Snack:

• Handful of walnuts.

Day 5:

Breakfast:

• Sliced turkey with tomato and avocado

Lunch:

• Chicken and vegetable stir-fry with broccoli, red bell peppers, and a tamari sauce

Dinner:

• Baked cod with roasted sweet potatoes and a side of sautéed spinach

Snack:

• Sliced cucumbers with tzatziki sauce

Day 6:

Breakfast:

• Scrambled eggs with sautéed kale and a side of fresh cherries

Lunch:

• Grilled shrimp and vegetable skewers with a side of quinoa

Dinner:

• Turkey meatballs with tomato sauce, served over spaghetti squash

Snack:

• Sliced pears with almond butter

Day 7:

Breakfast:

• Greek yogurt parfait with layers of walnuts, sliced strawberries, and honey

Lunch:

• Spinach and artichoke-stuffed chicken breast with a side salad

Dinner:

• Pan-seared halibut with steamed broccoli and a lemon-tarragon sauce

Snack:

• Celery sticks with guacamole

Day 8:

Breakfast:

• Scrambled eggs with spinach and a side of sliced plums

Lunch:

• Grilled chicken breast with a mixed green salad and a vinaigrette dressing

Dinner:

• Baked trout with roasted Brussels sprouts and a lemon-butter sauce

Snack:

• Sliced cucumbers with hummus

Day 9:

Breakfast:

• Greek yogurt with fresh blueberries and a drizzle of honey

Lunch:

• Turkey and avocado lettuce wraps with tomato and red onion

Dinner:

• Stir-fried lean beef with broccoli, ginger, and a tamari sauce, served over cauliflower rice

Snack:

• Sliced apples with almond butter

Day 10:

Breakfast:

• Omelette with mushrooms, red bell peppers, and a side of fresh cherries

Lunch:

• Spinach and kale salad with grilled shrimp, red onion, and olive oil dressing

Dinner:

• Roasted chicken thighs with steamed green beans and a garlic-herb seasoning

Snack:

• Carrot sticks with guacamole

Day 11:

Breakfast:

• Smoothie with almond milk, flaxseeds, mixed berries, and a scoop of protein powder

Lunch:

• Tuna salad with mixed greens, celery, and olive oil dressing

Dinner:

• Grilled lamb chops with a mint and garlic marinade, served with sautéed spinach

Snack:

• Handful of walnuts.

Day 12:

Breakfast:

• Sliced turkey with avocado and tomato

Lunch:

• Chicken and vegetable stir-fry with broccoli, red bell peppers, and a tamari sauce

Dinner:

• Baked cod with roasted sweet potatoes and a side of sautéed kale

Snack:

• Sliced pears with almond butter

Day 13:

Breakfast:

• Scrambled eggs with sautéed kale and a side of fresh plums

Lunch:

• Grilled shrimp and vegetable skewers with a side of quinoa

Dinner:

• Turkey meatballs with tomato sauce, served over spaghetti squash

Snack:

• Sliced celery with tzatziki sauce

Day 14:

Breakfast:

• Greek yogurt parfait with layers of walnuts, sliced strawberries, and honey

Lunch:

• Spinach and artichoke-stuffed chicken breast with a side salad

Dinner:

• Pan-seared halibut with steamed broccoli and a lemon-tarragon sauce

Snack:

• Sliced cucumbers with hummus

Supplement List For Blood Type O

Supplements can be an important component of the Blood Type Diet, designed to provide individuals with specific nutrients that may be lacking in their regular diet. While it's always best to obtain essential nutrients from whole foods, supplements can be a useful addition, especially if an individual's blood type diet restricts certain food groups or if there are specific health concerns.

Blood Type O Supplement List

For individuals with blood type O, the following supplements are recommended to support their nutritional needs:

1. Vitamin K: Vitamin K is crucial for blood clotting and bone health. Blood Type O individuals can benefit from vitamin K supplements, especially if they have a limited intake of leafy greens.

2. Probiotics: A healthy gut is essential for overall well-being, and probiotics can help maintain digestive health. Probiotic supplements can be particularly beneficial for people with type O blood.

3. Folate: Folate (vitamin B9) is important for DNA synthesis and repair, and it plays a role in preventing neural tube defects. Folate supplements can be beneficial, especially for pregnant blood type O women.

4. L-tyrosine: L-tyrosine is an amino acid that supports brain health and mood. It can be taken as a supplement by individuals with blood type O to support their mental and emotional well-being.

5. Calcium: Calcium is vital for bone health, and some blood type O individuals may benefit from calcium supplements, especially if they are not consuming dairy products.

6. Magnesium: Magnesium is important for muscle and nerve function, blood glucose control, and bone health. Blood Type O individuals can consider magnesium supplements if their diet lacks magnesium-rich foods.

7. Bromelain: Bromelain is an enzyme found in pineapple that can aid in digestion and reduce inflammation. Blood Type O individuals can take bromelain supplements to support their digestive health.

8. Ginger: Ginger supplements can help with digestion, reduce inflammation, and support the immune system. Blood Type O individuals may find ginger particularly beneficial.

9. Turmeric: Turmeric contains curcumin, which has anti-inflammatory and antioxidant properties. Turmeric supplements can help maintain overall health for people with type O blood.

10. Coenzyme Q10 (CoQ10): CoQ10 is involved in energy production and can benefit heart health. It can be considered by blood type O individuals to support their cardiovascular system.

Supplement Considerations

Before incorporating supplements into your diet, it's essential to consult with a healthcare professional, such as a doctor or registered dietitian. They can help you determine which supplements are appropriate for your specific needs and ensure they won't interact with any medications you may be taking.

Supplements should complement a balanced diet rather than replace it. It's important to remember that while supplements can be beneficial, whole foods remain the primary source of essential nutrients.

CHAPTER 13

*Beyond the Diet: Exercise
and Lifestyle*

While the Blood Type O Diet focuses on dietary recommendations, a holistic approach to health and well-being extends beyond food choices. Exercise and lifestyle play a crucial role in promoting overall health and vitality for individuals with blood type O. In this discussion, we will delve into exercise recommendations, adopting a healthy and balanced lifestyle, stress management, and relaxation techniques tailored to the needs of Blood Type O individuals.

Exercise Recommendations for Blood Type O Individuals:

1. Vigorous Physical Activity: Blood Type O individuals are often encouraged to engage in vigorous physical activities. These activities can include high-intensity interval training, cardiovascular exercises, and strength training. Engaging in regular workouts can help maintain a healthy weight, improve cardiovascular health, and enhance overall fitness.

2. Aerobic Exercise: Aerobic exercises, such as running, swimming, or cycling, are beneficial for blood type O individuals. These activities help improve oxygen circulation, boost metabolism, and enhance cardiovascular health.

3. Strength Training: Incorporating strength training exercises, such as weightlifting or bodyweight workouts, can help build and maintain lean muscle mass. This can aid in weight management and improve metabolic efficiency.

4. Flexibility and Balance: Blood Type O individuals should not overlook flexibility and balance exercises, such as yoga and Pilates. These activities promote joint health, reduce the risk of injury, and enhance overall well-being.

5. Consistency: Consistency is key. Blood Type O individuals should strive for a regular exercise routine, ideally 3-5 times a week, to maximize the benefits of physical activity.

Adopting a Healthy and Balanced Lifestyle:

1. Adequate Sleep: Prioritize a consistent sleep schedule, aiming for 7-9 hours of quality sleep per night. Quality sleep supports physical and mental recovery, making it an essential component of overall health.

2. Hydration: Stay well-hydrated by drinking plenty of water throughout the day. Adequate hydration is vital for maintaining energy levels and overall health.

3. Mindful Eating: Beyond food choices, how you eat matters. Adopt mindful eating practices by eating slowly, savoring your food, and paying attention to hunger and fullness cues.

4. Portion Control: Be mindful of portion sizes to prevent

overeating and maintain a healthy weight.

5. Stress Reduction: Chronic stress can impact the health of blood type O individuals. Practice stress-reduction techniques, such as deep breathing, meditation, or mindfulness, to manage stress effectively.

6. Social Connections: Foster positive social connections and engage in activities that bring joy and a sense of community. Social support can improve mental and emotional well-being.

Stress Management and Relaxation Techniques:

1. Meditation: Regular meditation practice can help reduce stress, improve focus, and promote emotional well-being. Techniques like mindfulness meditation can be particularly beneficial.

2. Deep Breathing: Incorporate deep breathing exercises into your daily routine. Deep, diaphragmatic breathing can calm the nervous system and reduce stress.

3. Yoga: Yoga combines physical activity, mindfulness, and relaxation. It can improve flexibility, reduce stress, and enhance overall wellness.

4. Hobbies and Recreation: Engaging in hobbies and recreational activities that bring joy and relaxation can help reduce stress and provide an emotional outlet.

5. Professional Support: If stress and anxiety become overwhelming, consider seeking support from a mental health professional, such as a counselor or therapist, who can provide coping strategies and emotional support.

CONCLUSION

In conclusion, "Blood Type Diet & Cookbook: A Comprehensive Guide To Understanding What To Eat For Your Type With Blood Type O Food, Beverage, Healthy Recipes, And Supplement Lists" has provided a thorough exploration of the Blood Type O diet, offering valuable insights into how dietary choices can potentially impact the well-being of individuals with this blood type.

Throughout this book, we've delved into the origins and evolution of the Blood Type Diet, gaining an understanding of its creator and the concept of individualized nutrition based on blood type. We've explored the importance of a healthy diet in enhancing overall well-being, especially for those with blood type O, and gained insights into the characteristics and traits associated with blood type O individuals.

Additionally, we've examined the dietary principles, food recommendations, and sample recipes that align with the Blood Type O Diet, promoting a balanced and nutritious approach to eating. We've provided 14-day meal plans and an array of recipes to help individuals with blood type O make informed and health-conscious choices when planning their daily meals.

Beyond dietary recommendations, we've emphasized the significance of exercise and lifestyle choices, highlighting how physical activity, mindful eating, stress management, and relaxation techniques can further enhance health and vitality for Blood Type O individuals.

As we conclude this journey through the Blood Type O diet, it is essential to remember that this dietary approach is a guideline, and individual variations may exist. It is always advisable to consult with healthcare professionals or registered dietitians for personalized dietary recommendations tailored to your specific health needs and goals.

The journey towards improved health and well-being is ongoing, and this book has served as a valuable resource, equipping you with knowledge and practical tools to make informed choices. We hope it empowers you to embark on a path of health and vitality that aligns with your unique blood type, ultimately leading to a life filled with wellness and energy.

Thank you for joining us on this journey, and we wish you the very best on your path to a healthier, happier, and more vibrant you.